INTERPERSONAL SKILLS
FOR HEALTH PROFESSIONALS

INTERPERSONAL SKILLS
FOR HEALTH PROFESSIONALS

Brian A. Gerrard
PhD.
McMaster University

Wendy J. Boniface
R.N. M.H.Sc.
Yale University

Barbara H. Love
R.N. BSc.N. M.H.Sc.
McMaster University

Reston Publishing Company, Inc.
A Prentice-Hall Company
Reston, Virginia

Library of Congress Cataloging in Publication Data

Gerrard, Brian.
  Interpersonal skills for health professionals.

  Bibliography: p.
  Includes index.
  1. Medical personnel and patient.   2. Interpersonal relations.   I. Boniface, Wendy, joint
author.   II. Love, Barbara, 1948–   joint author.
III. Title.   [DNLM: 1. Health occupations.
2. Interpersonal relations.   W62 G378i]
R727.3.G45   610.69'6   80-13470

ISBN 0-8359-3138-2
ISBN 0-8359-3136-6 (pbk.)

© 1980 by
Reston Publishing Company, Inc.
A Prentice-Hall Company
Reston, Virginia, 22090

10   9   8   7   6   5   4   3   2   1

Printed in the United States of America

To Florence, Jim, and Tony

CONTENTS

Foreword

Recent years have seen a mounting awareness of the connection between behavior, physical illness, recovery, and well being. Mode of life has emerged as a major pathogen: There is, now, little doubt of the place of maladaptive behavior in the etiology of many common and serious disorders. These disorders crowd the consulting rooms of practitioners and of clinics; they swell health budgets; and they have remained obdurately resistant to many well-intentioned administrative strategems.

In a more positive vein, the behavioral sciences have come of age in relation to medicine. The term *Behavioral Medicine* is gaining acceptance to denote the application of the theory and practice of the behavioral sciences to the theory and practice of modern medicine. Much has recently emerged in the areas of the psychology of communication, learning theory, cognitive appraisal, attitude, and motivation to suggest that these areas, all involving interpersonal skills, have a great deal to offer in helping patients to assume a more active and informed role in understanding the antecedents of their illness, the disease process itself, and the management of their own recovery and subsequent life style routines. Communication is at the very heart of a Health Care Team. The root of the term is significant: communication (from the Latin *communicare*) implies sharing; sharing of knowledge and of responsibility.

Implicit in the above is the central place of interpersonal skills in the provision of health care—be it in the planning or delivery; in actual case management in an institutional setting, or office, or home; in preventive counselling, or continued aftercare, and rehabilitation. Good interpersonal skills can be profoundly therapeutic. They enhance trust; they promote a partnership between an informed provider and an equally informed consumer. In a health care team, they favor cooperation rather than competition, sharing rather than divisiveness, coordination rather than wasteful overlap, and a win/win rather than a win/lose solution. They promote a Systems approach to health care. Systems, like Trust, are indivisible; and the "whole" of health care clearly amounts to more than a sum of its parts.

There is, fortunately, a steadily lessening mystique about interpersonal skills. In fact, it is becoming quite apparent that they can be codified, taught, and learned. The authors of this book have rendered the health field a great and practical service by defining needs in relevant areas, codifying resources, and describing training approaches. They have addressed these in relation to team functioning, individual coping, facilitation, problem-solving, and an objective appraisal of skill acquisition. Furthermore, their approach is significant in another respect, namely, their insistence, from the beginning, on an *experiential* approach to learning. The book is both Text and Workbook. Scholarship is conjoined with practical instances and case vignettes, which highlight issues and difficulties one encounters in practice. The authors, thus, not only impart a body of knowledge, derived from rich personal experience, but convey an attitude. Their practical, positive pragmatism should appeal to health professionals both in training and in practice, no matter what the terrain.

The book, thus, is timely. It meets a need. It is my personal hope, expressed to the authors, that it may mark the mere beginning of a continued endeavor in the future education of health professionals.

Joel Elkes, M.D.
Professor, Department of Psychiatry
McMaster University
Distinguished Service Professor, Emeritus
The Johns Hopkins University

How To Use This Book

This book shows you how to develop basic interpersonal skills that will help you to become a more effective health professional. It is a book for students, instructors, and practicing health professionals. It is meant for physicians, nurses, occupational therapists, physiotherapists, medical technicians, dentists, para-professionals— all professionals involved in the delivery of health care.

The interpersonal skills described are useful for coping effectively with common interpersonal problems experienced by all health professionals: distressed patients, aggressive patients, team conflict, and interpersonal stress. You can also use these skills to facilitate your problem-solving with patients or in teams. There is experimental evidence that the interpersonal skills taught in this book promote a trusting relationship with patients that produces a variety of positive physiological, psychological, and behavioral gains for patients.

This book presents a skill-oriented approach to learning basic interpersonal skills that aid health professionals in the delivery of health care. In addition to describing different interpersonal skills, this book gives clinical examples of how each interpersonal skill can be used and provides detailed worksheets and exercises that will assist you in actually learning specific interpersonal skills.

Chapter 1: WHY HEALTH PROFESSIONALS NEED INTER-PERSONAL SKILLS presents the rationale for the entire book. It describes in theoretical terms why interpersonal skills are useful for health professionals, and it presents research evidence for the effectiveness of, and the need for, interpersonal skills for health professionals.

Chapter 2: DEVELOPING SKILLS IN UNDERSTANDING INTERPERSONAL BEHAVIOR describes four useful models of interpersonal behavior that will help you to understand your interactions with patients and other health professionals.

Chapter 3: DEVELOPING SKILLS FOR COPING WITH INTERPERSONAL STRESS tells you how to "stress inoculate" yourself so that you don't become overstressed by the everyday demands of your job as a health professional. Being exposed to stress is part of being a health professional. If you find that you sometimes get so stressed by patients or other health professionals that you have difficulty carrying out your job, this chapter will show you how to reduce your stress to manageable levels so that you can function effectively.

Chapter 4: DEVELOPING FACILITATION SKILLS describes in step-by-step fashion how to go about developing a relationship of trust with your patients and colleagues. In this chapter, you will learn how to develop your skills in WARMTH and in ACTIVE LISTENING. Research indicates that these two interpersonal skills promote a variety of positive outcomes in patients.

Chapter 5: DEVELOPING SKILLS IN BEHAVIOR CHANGE presents the essential principles of behavior change—principles that you can use to help your patients overcome personal problems that interfere with their health care. In this chapter, you will also learn ways of implementing constructive change in health care teams in order to reduce team conflict and increase the quality of patient care.

Chapter 6: DEVELOPING ASSERTION SKILLS tells you how to handle aggressive patients. The assertion skills you learn in this chapter can also be used to help you resolve conflict situations with other health professionals. The term *assertion* is sometimes confused with aggression. Assertion has nothing to do with aggression. *Assertion* is a synonym for interpersonal competence. The assertion skills you learn in this chapter will help you to become a more effective health professional.

Chapter 7: DEVELOPING SKILLS IN PROBLEM-SOLVING describes interpersonal skills you can use to solve interpersonal problems that block individual and team effectiveness. You will learn how to approach a problem creatively and how to avoid the pitfalls that block finding solutions to problems.

Chapter 8: DEVELOPING SKILLS IN UNDERSTANDING GROUP, TEAM, AND ORGANIZATIONAL BEHAVIOR describes basic concepts that will help you to understand how processes in small and large groups can affect your work as a health professional.

Chapter 9: DEVELOPING SKILLS IN ASSESSING INTERPERSONAL SKILLS tells you why, and how, to assess the interpersonal skills taught in this book. If you really want to find out whether you've learned the interpersonal skills you've been practicing, this chapter will show you how.

In order to learn an interpersonal skill described in this book, there are three steps you can follow. First, read the description of the interpersonal skill. This tells you what it is you have to do to demonstrate the skill. Second, read the examples provided. These will give you a feeling for what the skill looks like in action—as used with an actual patient or on a health care team. Third, complete the exercises that have been designed to help you identify and practice the skill. The last step is the most important one. You can't learn an interpersonal skill unless you practice it. This principle is nicely summarized by a saying attributed to Confucius:

> I hear and I forget
> I see and I remember
> I do and I understand

By practicing the interpersonal skills described in this book, you will learn them. And having learned them, you will become a more effective health professional.

Acknowledgments

As authors we owe a debt to those persons who have made a difference in our lives. They have helped us by demonstrating in their relationships with us the facilitating interpersonal skills we have written about. They have encouraged us directly and indirectly in our writing, teaching, and research on interpersonal skills.

We thank the following persons at McMaster University: Molly Anderson, Mary Blum-Devor, Jay Browne, Regina Browne, Mary Buzzell, Marie Dafoe, Joel Elkes, Cathy Fenton, Joseph Jacobs, Janice Kennett, Shirley Krochuk, Angus MacMillan, Alba Mitchell, Patrick Mohide, Vic Neufeld, Ruth Pallister, Vince Rudnick, Jack Sibley, Peter Tugwell, and Robin Weir. We thank David Abbey, Cliff Christensen, Lynn Davie, Mary-Alice Guttman, John Weiser, and Jeri Wine at the Ontario Institute for Studies in Education, University of Toronto; and Marg Csapo, William Gray, John Friesen, and Will Schwahn at the University of British Columbia. We owe special thanks also to Barbara Davies, Elizabeth "Betsy" Smith, Bob Cowling, and Sue Tait.

We also thank the members of our families for their support: Anthony Bellissimo, Helen and James Love, Catherine Love, Susan Love, Rakash Kumar, the Fibison, Canty, and Boniface families, Alex and Naomi Gerrard, and Patricia Gerrard.

Finally, we would like to thank Ben Wentzell, David Culverwell, and Diane Anderson at Reston for their helpful suggestions.

1

Why Health Professionals
Need Interpersonal Skills

A. INTERPERSONAL SKILLS AND HEALTH PRACTICE

Interpersonal skills are those skills which promote a good relationship between individuals. The health professional needs these skills to effectively establish a helping relationship with his patients. Possessing knowledge about patient conditions is not in itself sufficient for providing optimal care. For example, a health professional may know what type of historical information is needed from the patient. Unless this knowledge is coupled with good interpersonal skills though, the subsequent questioning may anger or threaten the patient. It is not uncommon for a patient who feels angered or threatened by questioning to respond by giving incomplete or incorrect answers. When poor interpersonal skills result in this type of interaction, the purpose for seeking out the health professional in the first place may be defeated.

History-taking is but one component of patient care. Completing a physical examination, giving information, planning therapy, and counseling are examples of other components. The effective health professional uses his interpersonal skills to supplement, and to enhance, his clinical skills.

Direct patient care is one aspect of a health care practice. The ability to relate well to colleagues, other professionals, and groups is another important aspect of providing service. Many problems arise that require a joint or group effort for finding a solution. One needs to be able to express an opinion, request information and respond appropriately to confrontation. These interpersonal skills, along with others, are necessary if the health professional is to facilitate the problem-solving process.

B. HOW DO HEALTH PROFESSIONALS VIEW INTERPERSONAL SKILLS?

All types of health professionals—dentists, physical therapists, nurses, occupational therapists, physicians—consider interpersonal skills important. A review of the literature shows that health professionals consider interpersonal skills valuable for a variety of reasons. Kimball (1970), Balint (1971), and Klein (1974) have stressed the importance of interpersonal skills for data-gathering and formulating a correct diagnosis. Dye (1963) conducted a study which demonstrated the importance of having the nurse find out how a patient feels, what the patient thinks he needs, and whether the patient feels he has been helped:

> Without such explorations, only five out of 14 patients studied in a medical-surgical unit could tell the nurse why they were in distress adequately enough for her to determine the nursing care they needed (p. 56).

Interpersonal skills are viewed as important for promoting patient confidence in the health professional's skills (Ben-Sira, 1976; Ware and Snyder, 1975); for establishing patient trust (Goldin and Russel, 1969); for reducing patient resistance to therapy and management (Smiley and Smiley, 1974); for increasing patient satisfaction (Korsch and Negrete, 1972; Aluise, 1977); for giving a clear explanation of his illness to a patient (Skipper, Tagliacozzo, and Mauksch, 1964); for aiding patient catharsis and tension release (Klein, 1974; Worby and Babineau, 1974); for avoiding negative non-verbal communication with patients (Eldred, 1960); for promoting patient problem-solving through acceptance of the patient's feelings (Klein, 1974; Kimbail, 1970); and for promoting the physical recovery of patients (Jourard, 1960).

Several authors identify interpersonal skills for health professionals as valuable for counseling (Kowalewski, 1972; Parkes, 1973; Kiely, 1971; Kales and Kales, 1975). Kowalewski (1972) has stated:

> If a physician does not counsel his patients, he should not be practicing (p. 32).

The type of counseling Kowalewski recommends physicians do is mainly developmental, such as pre-school counseling, pre-obesity counseling, premarital counseling, and pre-retirement counseling.

Other authors (Loch, 1972; Kiely, 1971; Korsch and Negrete, 1972) have stressed the importance of interpersonal skills vis-a-vis the psychosomatic nature of most illnesses.

> ... more than half of a physician's working time in patient care, particularly in fields such as general practice, pediatrics and internal medicine, is spent on problems involving primarily psychological factors and the need for communication rather than technical knowledge (Korsch and Negrete, 1972, p. 66).

Pavlou, Hartings, and Davis (1978); Mettlin and Woelfel (1975); and Pearlin (1978) have acknowledged the importance of the health professional's interpersonal skills for aiding patient coping in situations of stress that exacerbate disease. Health professionals use interpersonal skills to cope with difficult patients (Kimball, 1970; Shocker, 1973) and to cope with staff conflict (Jackson, 1959). In addition, health professionals consider interpersonal skills valuable for working with specific groups of patients, such as the aged (Bloom, 1971; Davidson, 1975), lung cancer patients (Brown, Wilkins, Buxton, and Abse, 1975), dying patients (Heyman, 1974), the bereaved (Irwin and Meier, 1973; Hampe, 1975), the adolescent (Orvin, 1970), the retarded (Kelly and Menolascino, 1975), parents of infants with Down's syndrome (Pueschel and Murphy, 1975), patients who are divorcing (Schmidt and Messner, 1975), the chronically ill (Sorenson and Amis, 1976), and young children (Wu, 1965).

C. THE RELATIONSHIP OF HEALTH PROFESSIONALS' INTERPERSONAL SKILLS TO PATIENT OUTCOME INDICES

The critical test of interpersonal skills for health professionals is whether they have a tangible effect on patient outcome indices. Patient outcome indices are typically of three types: psychological (e.g., patient satisfaction), physiological (e.g., changes in pulse rate, length of recovery time) and behavioral (e.g., compliance).

One of the most widely cited studies which relates the physician's interpersonal skills to patient compliance is that conducted by Korsch and Negrete (1972). This was a correlational study of 800 mothers of pediatric patients and their doctors. The interaction between doctor, patient, and patient's mother was assessed using Bales' Interaction Process Analysis. This interaction was related to the mother's perception of the visit as assessed by a post-visit interview and to the outcome measures of compliance, reassurance, and satisfaction as assessed by a follow-up interview. This study is significant because it is the largest study in which doctor-patient interaction was objectively measured using IPA.

Some of the findings were the following. First, the length of interaction between physician and mother did not affect the mother's satisfaction with her visit. This is significant in view of the complaint made by some health professionals that they do not have the time to practice good interpersonal skills. Second, 53.4% of the highly satisfied mothers complied with the physician's instructions, whereas only 16.7% of the highly dissatisfied patients did so. Third, 86% of the mothers who mentioned they liked the physician's communications skills were satisfied, whereas only 25% of the mothers who said they disliked the physician's communication skills were satisfied.

Other studies that report a significant positive correlation between compliance and patient satisfaction are Becker, Drachman, and Kirscht (1972); Kincey, Bradshaw, and Ley (1975); and Ludy, Gagnon, and Caiola (1977).

Liptak, Hulka, and Cassel (1977) studied 42 physicians and their interaction with 479 infants and their mothers. Significant findings were positive correlations between: physician awareness of maternal concerns and mother-child adaptation, physician communication to mother and mother's satisfaction, and physician management and mother's satisfaction. Ben-Sira (1976) found that, if the physician is friendly and caring towards his patient, the patient assumes the physician is skilled. Since patients have no clear criteria by which to judge the physician's clinical skills, it would appear that they assess the physician in terms of his interpersonal skills.

There is evidence that the health professional's interpersonal skills make a difference in the quality of care rendered to patients. A review of 27 studies using control groups found that, out of 98 outcome assessments made, 62 (63%) demonstrated the occurrence of beneficial physiological, psychological, or behavioral changes in patients (Gerrard, 1978). In view of the fact that there was minimal replication in these studies, with few studies using the same outcome measure, and many of the treatment effects appeared weak, the finding that 24 out of the 27 studies (89%) had positive patient outcomes for the interpersonal skills treatment suggests—at the very least—a moderate relationship between health professionals' interpersonal skills and patient outcome. It seems clear that the health professional's interpersonal skills improve patient coping with and recovery from disease, although the extent of this improvement must be determined by further research.

D. DO HEALTH PROFESSIONALS LACK INTERPERSONAL SKILLS?

Health professionals do consider interpersonal skills valuable and it has been shown that they affect patient outcomes. Do health professionals have these skills? Numerous writers (Cline and

Garrard, 1973; Elstein, Kagan, and Shulman, 1972; Froelich, 1969; Jason, Kagan, Werner, Elstein, and Thomas, 1970; Moreland, Ivey, and Phillips, 1973; Pacoe, Naar, Guyett, and Wells, 1976; Rasche, Bernstein, and Veen Huis, 1974; Secundy and Katz, 1975; Taylor and Berven, 1974; Waldon, 1973; Werner and Schneider, 1974) have pointed out that interpersonal skills do not come naturally to health professionals and that health professionals must receive explicit skills training in order to master interpersonal skills. This conclusion is supported by Ware, Strassman, and Naftulin (1971) who found that, for a group of 62 medical students, there was a negative relationship between understanding interviewing principles and interview performance. Even if medical students are given explicit training by specialized staff in interpersonal skills, the failure of other important medical staff to model these skills may have a negative effect on students' interpersonal skills (Scott, Donnelly, and Hess, 1976; Santiesteban, 1975). Helfer (1970) has reported that, as the student moves through his years in medical school, his interpersonal skills tend to decline. There is some evidence that, as length of practice increases, nurses tend to lose empathic ability (Forsyth, 1977). It is possible that health professionals, although initially trained to satisfactory levels of interpersonal skills, lose their skills through exposure to significant role models who do not model a high level of interpersonal skills.

Further evidence that health professionals lack interpersonal skills comes from surveys on patient dissatisfaction with health professionals, studies measuring health professionals' interpersonal skills, and surveys of interpersonal problems experienced by health professionals.

Patient surveys show that from 5% to 96% of patients are dissatisfied with the communication they have with health professionals. The studies and percentages of patients complaining about communication are shown in Table 1.1.

Other studies reporting patient dissatisfaction with health professionals are Ley and Spelman (1967), Duff and Hollingshead (1968), Smith (1969), and Ujhely (1974).

Probably the best known study of health professionals using direct assessment of interpersonal skills was made by the previously mentioned Korsch and Negrete (1972). It was found that 76% of the mothers were satisfied overall with their visits. However, 19% of the mothers felt they had received no clear statement of what was wrong with their baby, and almost half were unsure of what had caused their child's illness.

The absence of an explanation of the cause is unnerving in such a situation, because the mother of a sick baby generally has a tendency to blame herself for the occurrence and needs specific reassurance (Korsch and Negrete, 1972, p. 69).

TABLE 1.1:   PATIENTS COMPLAINING ABOUT COMMUNICATION WITH HEALTH PROFESSIONALS.

Study	Percentage of patients complaining about communication with health professionals
McGhie (1961)	65%
Hetherington, et al. (1963)	54%
Cartwright (1964)	29%
Jones, et al. (1964)	39%
Houghton (1968)	35%
Raphael (1969)	18%
United Manchester Hospitals (1970)	5-17%
Raphael (1967)	42%
Carstairs (1970)	79-96%

In more than half the cases recorded, the physician used medical jargon. Civilities, such as introducing themselves or addressing each other by name, occurred infrequently. Twenty-six percent of the mothers told the interviewers after their visit with the physician that they had not told their greatest concern to the physician because they were not encouraged to do so or did not have an opportunity to do so.

A frequent cause of dismay for the mother was the physician's total disregard of her account of what chiefly worried her about her child's illness ... Some patients were so preoccupied with their dominant concern that they were unable to listen to the physician (Korsch and Negrete, 1972, p. 72).

Another study examined the interactions that occurred in a hospital setting. Using raters who observed ongoing hospital interactions, Krebs (1976) found that 6% of the total interactions were disrespectful and 34% were respectful. He concluded that, while the percentage of disrespectful interactions appeared small, it probably represented an excess of 100,000 disrespectful interactions occurring within the hospital each week. Krebs concluded that this quantity of disrespectful interactions, plus the fact that anyone involved in or observing an example of disrespect is not likely to forget it quickly, was having a signficiant impact on the hospital he was studying.

Surveys of interpersonal problems experienced by health professionals also give evidence that they lack interpersonal skills. Sethee (1967) surveyed a sample of 30 nurses and found that 70% found emotion-laden situations difficult to deal with. Some of the difficulties encountered were: passive patients, feeling inadequate in knowing how to assess the situation and knowing how to respond, and feeling uncomfortable during silences. Davitz (1972) found that the greatest cause of stress for 37 nursing students in a Nigerian school of nursing was critical evaluation of their performance, followed by patient hostility, and problems in interpersonal relationships with other staff. Stein (1969) surveyed 108 nursing students in order to identify dominant areas of concern and conflict in caring for patients. Some of the problem areas, and the percentage of nurses identifying each problem area as troublesome, were: not enough communication with physicians about patient's welfare (92.6%); too much authority by physicians, lack of respect for nursing reports and judgments (62%); dealing with the death of a patient (56.5%); deciding how to answer a patient's questions when there is no known cure (80.6%); making mistakes in nursing practice (86.1%); too much impersonality of patient care and neglect of their emotional needs (79.6%); feeling frustrated that I can't do more for my patients to make them more comfortable (82.4%); caring for a patient who will not accept my teaching (76.9%); and dealing with anxious patients and those with emotional outbursts (57.4%).

Coburn and Jovaisas (1975) surveyed 52 first year medical students for current and anticipated sources of stress. The top four current sources of stress all relate to worries about academic performance. The top three anticipated sources of stress are: death of a patient, fear of error in diagnosis or treatment, and dealing with a patient with a chronic and helpless disease. MacNamara (1974) found that the main problems encountered by medical students were: marital/sexual topics, how to reassure and interview patients, dying patients, making a mistake, uncooperative or hostile patients, and silence.

These surveys of problems experienced by medical and nursing students show that the three most difficult problems faced by students are aggressive patients, making mistakes/being evaluated, and dying patients. In addition, nurses experience problems in being assertive with physicians, and medical students have anxieties about discussing marital and sexual problems with patients. Although these surveys do not provide any direct evidence for physicians and nurses lacking interpersonal skills, they identify areas for which any lack of interpersonal skills would tend to produce a "problem area" for the health professional.

Studies of nurses have reported conflict with physicians and sexist attitudes towards nurses in intensive care and critical care units (Robinson, 1972); lack of belonging and poor professional communication in health care teams (Warren, 1978); general conflict in the nurse-physician relationship due to physician attitudes of sexism and classism (Hoekelman, 1975); and conflict between residents and experienced nurses resulting from residents' anxiety (Sabshin, 1957). These four studies are of interest because they focus on interpersonal problems at the team level.

"Problem" patients that health professionals have difficulty coping with are patients who are: dying (Quint, 1966; Feifel, 1967; Kubler-Ross, 1970; Nelson, 1973; Lester, Getty and Kneisl, 1974; Fairchild, 1977; Cassileth, 1978), crying (Norris, 1957; Knowles, 1959; Robinson, 1968; Forster and Forster, 1971), aggressive—this includes the following aggressive patient roles: the demander, the threatener, abusive, insensitive, the help rejector, the manipulator—(Himmelhock, Davies, Tucker, and Alderman, 1970; Nelson, 1973; Scoggins, 1976; Katz, 1978), mentally ill (Nelson, 1973), hypochondriacs (Nelson, 1973; Katz, 1978), and over-dependent (Katz, 1978).

"Unpopular" patients that health professionals tend to dislike, and therefore withhold use of their interpersonal skills with, are: the chronically ill (Stockwell, 1972; Nelson, 1973), foreign patients (Stockwell, 1972), patients with physical defects (Stockwell, 1972), and the elderly (Miller, Brimigion, Keller, and Woodruff, 1972). There is some evidence that "problem" and "unpopular" patients receive poorer quality care than more popular patients (Lorber, 1975; Spitzer and Sobel, 1962). Spitzer and Sobel (1962) suggest that, when a health professional lacks the interpersonal skills to collect sufficient data from a patient or to cope with an upset patient, he feels frustrated, helpless, and anxious. The health professional responds to this anxiety by displacing his feelings onto the patient as dislike.

> A circular pattern is evolved which is difficult to break and which may have a dysfunctional effect on the quality of care received by that patient, on his rate of improvement, and on the relationships between the members of the hospital staff (p. 235).

In summary, this review of the literature suggests that many health professionals do lack interpersonal skills. The main interpersonal problems that health professionals seem to have difficulty handling are: distressed patients (who are upset, in pain, crying, etc.), aggressive patients, team conflict, evaluation anxiety (i.e., anxiety about being evaluated; fear of making a mistake), and unappealing patients. The literature indicates that many health professionals experience a great deal of stress when they encounter these five interpersonal problem areas. If a health professional lacks the interpersonal skills to handle these interpersonal problem areas, his stress may become so great that it affects his quality of care. This should be a matter of serious concern to all health professionals.

E.   INTERPERSONAL SKILLS IN PRACTICE

There are three basic types of interpersonal problems that health professionals have to deal with:

1. Situations in which the patient has a problem which is upsetting him and preventing him from focusing on a task (e.g., obese patient cries because she feels she'll never lose weight);

2. Situations in which a health professional and a patient work together to complete a task (e.g., working together to plan a diet that is medically sound and acceptable to the patient);

3. Situations in which a health professional has a problem responding to another person's behavior (e.g., health professional stressed because he does not know how to handle a crying patient).

There are different types of interpersonal skills that are useful in each of these areas. The diagram on page 11 illustrates this.* FACILITATION SKILLS and BEHAVIOR CHANGE SKILLS are the interpersonal skills which are used when the patient has a problem which prevents him from working on a task. PROBLEM-SOLVING INTERPERSONAL SKILLS are those which are used

---

* The diagram is an adaptation of one used by Thomas Gordon in his book: *T.E.T. TEACHER EFFECTIVENESS TRAINING*, New York: Wyden, 1974.

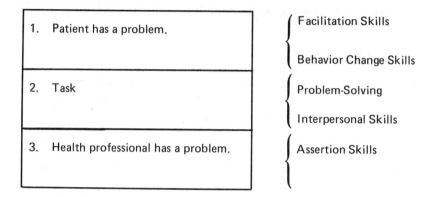

DIAGRAM 1.1

to accomplish a task efficiently. ASSERTION SKILLS are inter-personal skills which are used to handle a situation in which the health professional has a problem.

1.   Patient Has A Problem

This represents the patient who has a problem and seeks help. The health professional has a responsibility to identify and understand the patient's complaint, not only in terms of the health-illness continuum but also in terms of the patient's perception of his problem, his conflicts and fears. Facilitation skills and behavior change skills (e.g., interpretation, reframing, and behavior modifi-cation) assist the health professional in identifying patient prob-lems, counseling, allaying anxiety, and in planning management that will have a therapeutic effect.

The following examples illustrate the value of facilitation skills and behavior change skills.

Example

Mrs. Barnes has brought 3-month-old Jon to her health professional for the second time in a month for a minor cold. It is her first baby, and he has been growing and developing very nicely. Today, while the health profes-sional takes a history of his illness, Mrs. Barnes nervous-ly rocks the baby, puts a bottle in and out of his mouth, burps him frequently, and repeatedly shifts Jon's posi-tion in her arms. Mrs. Barnes appears tense and upset.

The health professional completes the history and physical examination.

Dialogue A

Health professional: Jon looks fine. He has a slight cold. Clean his nose like we discussed during your last visit. Give him plenty of liquids and turn the vaporizer on.

Mrs. Barnes: Are you *sure* he's OK?

Health professional: (as she helps Mrs. Barnes to the waiting room) No need to worry! Call if he develops a fever or any new symptoms.

Mrs. Barnes looks close to tears as she dresses Jon in the waiting room.

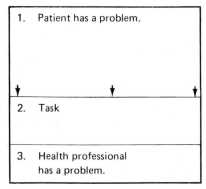

Mrs. Barnes is tense and upset!	1. Patient has a problem.	The health professional lacks FACILITATION SKILLS and is unable to reassure Mrs. Barnes.
She has less energy to devote to mothering tasks.	2. Task	
	3. Health professional has a problem.	

DIAGRAM 1.2

Dialogue B

Health professional: Jon has a slight cold but is otherwise fine. (SILENCE) You seem upset today, Mrs. Barnes. (ACTIVE LISTENING). Are you worried about something you haven't mentioned?

Mrs. Barnes: I try so hard to do everything right, but he keeps getting sick!

Health professional: Many women are very concerned about being good mothers and when their children get sick, they feel as if they've failed. Could this be how you're feeling?

Mrs. Barnes: Yes, it is. Have I done something wrong?

Health professional: No. In fact, you have been very conscientious about his care (ENCOURAGEMENT). Colds are caused by viruses, and we don't always know why some babies are more susceptible than others. We don't have a cure for the common cold, but I can tell you ways of making Jon more comfortable (INFORMATION-GIVING).

Mrs. Barnes looks visibly relieved and holds Jon quietly while the health professional continues with instructions for caring for the cold.

Discussion

In Dialogue A, the health professional identified the minor illness and gave information but was ineffective in allaying Mrs. Barnes' anxiety. It is not uncommon for a baby to respond to parental anxiety or tension with crying. It is easy to see the effect crying could have on a mother who is already feeling unsure of her mothering abilities. By not responding to Mrs. Barnes' behavior, the health professional missed an opportunity to be helpful to this family.

In Dialogue B, the health professional observed Mrs. Barnes' behavior and reflected this observation back to her, using a technique called ACTIVE LISTENING, and in this brief interchange was able to identify the real problem for this mother. The health

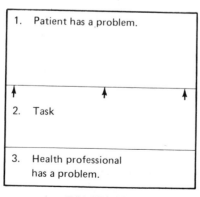

Mrs. Barnes is relieved.

She has more energy to devote to mothering tasks.

1. Patient has a problem.

2. Task

3. Health professional has a problem.

The health professional uses FACILITATION SKILLS to reassure Mrs. Barnes.

DIAGRAM 1.3

professional then gave ENCOURAGEMENT to Mrs. Barnes about her mothering abilities, and followed it with INFORMATION-GIVING. These helping skills made it possible for the health professional to effectively allay Mrs. Barnes anxiety.

Example

Mark is a student who is just beginning his clinical experience with patients. In his first week, he was assigned to a family practice unit where he was responsible for doing histories and physicals on patients of all ages for a variety of reasons. At the end of the week, he met with the health professional who was his instructor to review his experiences.

Dialogue A

Health professional: So, you've finished your first week. You've had some interesting cases. Is there anything more I can help you with? Do you have any questions?

Student: I think you answered most of my questions as they came up. I need to do some more reading on some of the specific conditions I saw. (Pause) There is an area I seem to be having difficulty with and that is the sexual history. It's such a sensitive topic for most people, and I find myself stuttering and tripping over my words. I feel as if I'm intruding. And when . . .

Health professional: Relax. It's just a stage. We all have to go through it. You'll learn. When it's indicated, just set your mind and do it. Is there anything else?

Student: I guess not. Could you give me that reference on blood pressure you mentioned earlier?

Dialogue B

Health professional: It's been a busy week! Is there anything more I can help you with? Do you have any questions?

Student: You answered most of my questions as they came up. I need to do some more reading on some of the specific conditions I saw. (Pause) There is an area I seem to be having difficulty with and that is the sexual history. It's such a sensitive topic for most people, and I find myself stuttering and tripping over my words. I feel as if it's none of my business.

Health professional: You're saying that you are uncomfortable taking a sexual history, and you feel as if you're intruding (ACTIVE LISTENING).

Student: That's right.

Health professional: I think that initial discomfort must be a universal feeling (REASSURANCE). When I first started taking sexual histories, my words were smooth, but I kept blushing (SELF-DISCLOSURE). I have learned that, by asking questions appropriately, you let patients know you are interested in helping them with this aspect of their health. Many patients, when given the opportunity, welcome a chance to ask questions or discuss concerns (REFRAMING). They may not do so at that particular visit, but the ground rules are set— you've identified yourself as a resource.

Student: It really helps to see it from a different perspective. It certainly makes sense. It also helps to know others feel uncomfortable at first. Thank you for discussing it with me.

Discussion

This is not an uncommon situation. MacNamara (1974) found that one of the main problems encountered by medical students was discussing sexual problems with patients. As future health professionals, they need assistance in handling this aspect of patient care. Other health professionals share this need as well.

In Dialogue A, the health professional effectively blocked communication. His initial comment, "Relax," implied that it was not an issue worth worrying about. Encouragements such as "everyone goes through this sooner or later" are rarely helpful in the immediate situation. They are off-putting and do not focus on how the experience may be affecting this particular individual. The student responded to the messages from the health professional and backed off. He had not been helped, and furthermore, he was left to ponder why the health professional could not discuss it with him in a more helpful way.

In Dialogue B, FACILITATION SKILLS and BEHAVIOR CHANGE SKILLS were used. Initially, the health professional ACTIVELY LISTENED and provided REASSURANCE and SELF-DISCLOSURE. He then used a BEHAVIOR CHANGE SKILL—REFRAMING—when he approached the problem from a patient's perspective. The student was then able to see the sexual history not as an intrusion but as a way of giving the patient an opportunity to discuss his concerns. The student was helped with his problem and also saw good interpersonal skills role modeled.

2.   The Task

There are many tasks that need to be accomplished by health professionals in order to care for a patient and his family. Initially, the patient problem should be clearly defined. Interpersonal skills facilitate looking at a problem from different perspectives so that the best solution can be found. After the goal is established, related tasks need to be identified, delegated to the appropriate staff members, and coordinated. Participation in accomplishing the tasks needs to be encouraged and conflict managed. Involved professional and non-professional staff need and deserve feedback. Ideally, evaluation of the outcome occurs. PROBLEM-SOLVING INTERPERSONAL SKILLS are necessary to engage successfully in the activities related to patient care whether the role played be that of leader, supervisor, or group member. ACTIVE LISTENING, CLARIFYING, and EXPRESSING AN OPINION are examples of skills that are valuable in accomplishing a task. When health professionals possess these skills, many positive outcomes result. Ideas and feelings are openly expressed. Staff are able to openly acknowledge strengths and weaknesses, so it becomes clear who can make what contribution to getting the task done. Social and system realities are established.

Example

Mr. Wendell, a 63-year-old laborer, was hospitalized for the first time with a fractured femur. On admission, a health professional casually mentioned that his blood pressure was up. As part of the hospital routine, his blood pressure was taken daily during his stay. On day two, Mr. Wendell complained of a headache that was relieved by pain medication but would return when the medication wore off. On day three, Mr. Wendell became demanding, pushing his call bell frequently and making a wide range of requests. The situation was discussed on day four during the morning team report.

Dialogue A

Health professional #1: Mr. Wendell is driving me crazy! He is forever pushing his call bell.

Team leader: I know. Just do your best to answer it and help him out. He should be ready for discharge and home care in a few days.

Health professional #2: His pain medication needs to be renewed and I'll do that today.

Dialogue B

Health professional #1: Mr. Wendell is driving me crazy! He is forever pushing his call bell.

Team leader: What bothers you about that? (CLARIFICATION)

Health professional #1: He really doesn't need me . . . he just asks for silly things that he could do for himself. I keep encouraging him to do things because he'll have to when he goes home in a few days.

Health professional #2: What does he say?

Health professional #1: Nothing really. He just looks at me.

Team leader: Do you think he might need you in a different way?

Health professional #2: What do you mean? (CLARIFICATION)

Team leader: Perhaps he's worried about something and is afraid to ask.

Health professional #2: I have felt that his headaches have been related to stress (EXPRESSING AN

	OPINION), but I assumed it was due to the accident. I will renew his pain medication today, but I think this matter needs to be pursued.
Health professional #1:	You're concerned that his headaches are related to stress (ACTIVE LISTENING). Do you have any ideas about how we might find out *what* the source of stress is?
Health professional #2:	(To the team leader) Perhaps on your morning rounds, you could ask him if there is anything that is concerning him that he hasn't mentioned, or that we haven't made possible for him to bring up.
Team leader:	That's a nice approach. I'll do it today.

The team leader reported the next day that Mr. Wendell was worried about his blood pressure. She had reassured him but felt that he would need more reassurance. Health professional #2 said that he would build that into his care plan when he saw Mr. Wendell as an outpatient.

Discussion

In Dialogue A, the team leader did not CLARIFY why the frequent patient calls were bothersome to the health professional, and consequently the real problem was not identified. Instead, the problem became the "demanding patient," and the solution rested in his discharge.

In Dialogue B, the team members demonstrated a variety of PROBLEM-SOLVING INTERPERSONAL SKILLS—CLARIFICATION, ACTIVE LISTENING, EXPRESSING AN OPINION—as they worked toward a solution. CLARIFICATION SKILLS assisted with problem identification. (Mr. Wendell was worried about his blood pressure.) ACTIVE LISTENING helped to draw out opinions and suggestions for handling the problem. The use of these skills resulted in two positive outcomes: the patient problem was solved (Mr. Wendell was reassured, and the frequent calling stopped) and the team leader increased her skills.

3. You Have the Problem

At times, the health professional finds himself in a situation where he is being put down, treated unfairly, or where unreasonable requests are being made of him. An inability to respond in a clear, direct, and open manner results in negative feelings, and the energy required to cope with these feelings is no longer available for accomplishing the task or solving the problem. For example, the health professional who cannot say "no" to unreasonable requests may become overwhelmed with work and soon begin to feel trapped and angry. He may react with aggressive behavior and blame others. The involved staff then react to the aggressive behavior with their own negative feelings. In this situation, energy available for constructive work is greatly reduced. Being able to say "no" to an unreasonable request, and being able to constructively confront aggressive patients or health professionals are two of the most important ASSERTION SKILLS health professionals need. They enable the health professional to respond promptly and directly. Messages are clear.

Example

The health professional had a full morning of patients booked. Mr. Thomas' 5-year-old daughter was scheduled for a ten-minute appointment to have stitches removed from her chin. After they were removed, Mr. Thomas handed the health professional a lengthy school physical form.

Mr. Thomas: Could you take care of this as well? It would save me a second trip.

Response A

Health professional: Well, I guess so.

The health professional felt used and stressed because there were patients waiting to be seen who were on time. He went home with a headache.

Response B

Health professional: If you insist!

The health professional approached the child in a brusque manner, and became impatient when the child refused to cooperate.

Health professional: (in a harsh voice) You'll have to learn to discipline your child better!

Discussion

Mr. Thomas asked the health professional to do a complete physical when the appointment had been for removal of two stitches. This was an unreasonable request in light of the health professional's schedule that day, and yet he was unable to say "no". Response A illustrates a NON-ASSERTIVE response. Outward behavior did not change, but the health professional felt stressed and angry. In Response B, the health professional became brusque and critical of the parent. This is an example of an AGGRESSIVE response. The diagram below shows that, in both examples, the health professional's inability to say "no" to an unreasonable request left him feeling stressed. The amount of energy required to cope with the stress was no longer available to devote to the task.

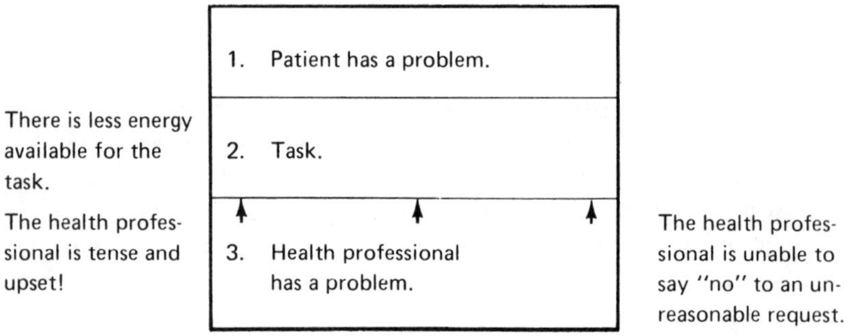

	1. Patient has a problem.	
There is less energy available for the task.	2. Task.	
The health professional is tense and upset!	3. Health professional has a problem.	The health professional is unable to say "no" to an unreasonable request.

DIAGRAM 1.4

Response C

Health professional: I would like to be able to save you a second trip, but we only scheduled a ten-minute appointment today for removal of stitches. Completing that form requires taking a more complete history and then a complete physical. I have other patients waiting to be seen, so it will not be possible to do it today. My secretary will be happy to schedule a time for next week.

Discussion

The health professional demonstrated an ASSERTION SKILL when he said "no" to an unreasonable request. He showed Mr.

Thomas respect by explaining why it was not possible to complete the form that day. This is important because patients are frequently unaware that they are making an unreasonable request. Saying "no" allowed the health professional to set a realistic limit on his work load and prevent feelings of anger and stress. It left more energy to devote to the task.

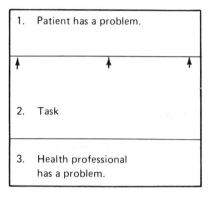

There is more energy to devote to the task.

The health professional does not become tense and upset.

The health professional used an ASSERTION SKILL and said "no" to an unreasonable request.

DIAGRAM 1.5

The following exercises are provided to give you an opportunity to apply your knowledge and to focus on your own interpersonal skills.

Exercise I: Where Is the Problem?

Purpose: To identify where the problem is that requires INTERPERSONAL SKILLS for solution.

Instructions: 1. Read the following vignettes and decide *where* the problem is;
2. In the space provided, describe *what* the problem is.

Situation A

Mrs. Hinds was hospitalized for abdominal surgery. The team leader was busy with an emergency and was not able to administer her pain medication before Mrs. Hinds had to get out of bed for the first time. Mrs. Hinds was very uncomfortable when the health professional helped her out of bed, and the experience left her feeling upset. A health professional on the evening shift went in to help Mrs. Hinds get out of bed a second time.

> *Mrs. Hinds*:   I won't get out of bed again today!
> *Health professional*:   It's ordered for you and you must.
> *Mrs. Hinds*:   I won't. You can just leave because coaxing won't work.
> *Health professional*:   Now, Mrs. Hinds . . .
> *Mrs. Hinds*:   Just get out of my room!

The health professional left the room.

WHERE IS THE PROBLEM?

- ☐ The patient has a problem.
- ☐ Task
- ☐ The health professional has a problem.

WHAT IS THE PROBLEM?

_____

_____

Situation B

A ward meeting was held to discuss changing the policy for visiting hours.

> *Group leader*:   We've had many requests to make the visiting hours longer.
> *Health professional #1*:   I'm not for it at all. It interrupts my work to always have visitors around. They don't like leaving the room when you need to do something for the patient.
> *Health professional #2*:   I know who you're remembering . . . the Durham family. (laugh) That was quite a crew.
> *Health professional #3*:   And then there was the Peck family.

The group members continued comparing experiences with families.

WHERE IS THE PROBLEM?

- ☐ The patient has a problem.
- ☐ Task
- ☐ The health professional has a problem.

WHAT IS THE PROBLEM?

Situation C

A health professional student was interviewing a patient in a specialty clinic in a small examining room. The patient was expressing her concern about her prognosis.

Patient: My disease seems to be progressing so fast. I'm really worried about my being able to take care of my family.

Student: When you find yourself thinking about next year, what . . . . .

A specialist new to the clinic opened the door without knocking, walked in and without introducing herself began:

Specialist: I've looked at the lab results, and they are the same as the last ones that were done.

The specialist continued to discuss the lab results and management plans.

WHERE IS THE PROBLEM?
- ☐ The patient has a problem.
- ☐ Task
- ☐ The health professional has a problem.

WHAT IS THE PROBLEM?

Situation D

An interdisciplinary group of health professionals from a large medical center was meeting weekly to set up a satellite pediatric clinic in a rural district.

Health professional #1:   We've been meeting now for three weeks. I think we should decide on

	what specific services we want to offer at the clinic.
Health professional #2:	I think what we should *first* decide is who will be going out there and then that will tell us what we can offer.
Health professional #3:	That's so limiting and short-sighted. We need some long range goals . . . We'll find the people and phase in the services gradually.
Health professional #2:	I can tell you've never been involved in a project like this before.
Health professional #3:	Have you?
Health professional #2:	Yes, several, and I know what happens.
Health professional #3:	What?
Health professional #2:	They go down the tubes unless you make plans around the resources you already have.
Health professional #4:	I think we should look at the budget and begin there. That will tell us what services we can afford.
Health professional #1:	The state has some ideas as a result of some research that was done in this area. The study supposedly identified some pressing needs.

Discussion continued like this.

WHERE IS THE PROBLEM?
- ☐ The patient has a problem.
- ☐ Task
- ☐ The health professional has a problem.

WHAT IS THE PROBLEM?

_____

_____

Answers to this exercise can be found in Appendix 1.

Exercise 2:   It Happened to Me

Purpose: To identify the need for INTERPERSONAL SKILLS.

Instructions: 1. (a) Briefly describe a situation you were involved in where the other person (patient/health professional) had a problem (felt upset).

_____

_____

(b) What INTERPERSONAL SKILLS were evident or lacking?

_____

2. (a) Briefly describe a situation you were involved in where you and another person had to accomplish a difficult task.

_____

_____

(b) What INTERPERSONAL SKILLS were evident or lacking?

_____

3. (a) Briefly describe a situation in which *you* had a problem (felt upset) because a patient or health professional was aggressive or made an unreasonable request of you.

_____

_____

(b) What INTERPERSONAL SKILLS were evident or lacking?

_____

4.   Share this in pairs.

Exercise 3:   Identifying Your Interpersonal Skills

Purpose: To develop skills in identifying your own strengths and weaknesses in INTERPERSONAL SKILLS.

Instructions: 1. Read each statement and then show the extent to which the statement applies to you by placing a check mark (✓) in the appropriate space to the right.

ALWAYS (A)
USUALLY (U)
SOMETIMES (S)
RARELY (R)
NEVER (N)

	A	U	S	R	N
1. I feel comfortable making a request when I need help.					
2. I am able to respond to a patient's feeling of sadness.					
3. I express my opinion in a group.					
4. I am able to help others see a situation in a different way.					
5. I am able to help a patient change an unhealthy pattern of living.					
6. I am at ease taking a psycho-social history from a patient.					
7. I am able to assist parents in changing their child's undesirable behavior.					
8. I say "no" when someone makes an unreasonable request of me.					
9. I show a patient I understand when he is upset.					
10. I give patients encouragement.					
11. I can defend my position without becoming aggressive.					
12. I ask colleagues to clarify statements that are ambiguous.					

2. Score your answers.

ALWAYS (A)   = 5
USUALLY (U)   = 4
SOMETIMES (S)   = 3
RARELY (R)   = 2
NEVER (N)   = 1

Add up your scores for questions 2, 9, 10.

_____
TOTAL

These are questions that focus on your FACILITATION SKILLS.

Add up your scores for questions 4, 5, 7.

_____
TOTAL

These are questions that focus on your BEHAVIOR CHANGE SKILLS.

Add up your scores for questions 3, 6, 12.

_____
TOTAL

These are questions that focus on your PROBLEM-SOLVING INTERPERSONAL SKILLS.

Add up your scores for questions 1, 8, 11.

_____
TOTAL

These are questions that focus on your ASSERTION SKILLS.

The highest score in any category is 15.
The lowest score in any category is 3.

SUMMARY

Interpersonal skills are skills that the health professional uses to develop a helping relationship with patients. The effective health professional uses interpersonal skills to supplement, and to enhance, clinical health care skills. Interpersonal skills facilitate better patient care by: reducing the health professional's stress; helping the health professional to understand why patients (and teams) act the way they do; developing a relationship of trust between health professional and patient; solving patients' personal problems that interfere with recovery; helping the health professional to constructively handle aggressive patients (and colleagues); stimulating the health professional to think of creative and effective solutions to interpersonal problems. Extensive research shows that interpersonal skills used by health professionals produce a variety of positive physiological, psychological, and behavioral outcomes for patients. Research also shows that health professionals tend to lack interpersonal skills and that they must be explicitly trained in order to acquire competence in these skills. The following chapters discuss in detail the interpersonal skills mentioned in this chapter.

2

Developing Skills In Understanding Interpersonal Behavior

A. WHAT IS
INTERPERSONAL BEHAVIOR?

Interpersonal behavior occurs between two or more persons: between a health professional and a patient, between a health professional and several patients (e.g., an interview with a mother and her child), or between several health professionals (e.g., at a team conference). The term "interpersonal" means "between persons." The term "behavior" refers to how a person behaves or acts, that is, what he says and does.

The concept of interpersonal behavior is important because research has shown that how one person behaves in a conversation with another person depends to a large extent upon who that other person is and how he behaves. It would be ideal if all a health professional had to do was to take a history from his patient and then initiate the appropriate therapy that would make the patient better. After all, isn't that what health care is all about—helping patients? But patients *and* health professionals have emotions, needs, beliefs, and values. They are not machines that function in a simple fashion. Your emotions, needs, beliefs, and values affect how you respond to your patients and how they, in turn, respond to you.

Example

A health professional is interviewing a new patient and the following conversation takes place.

Health professional: Take these pills for a week and then come back and see me.

Patient: What are these pills for? Could you tell me more about what they're supposed to do and any side effects they might have?

Health professional: (Getting angry) Look, if you don't trust me then perhaps you should go see another health professional.

Patient: (Getting angry) Well, maybe I should!

As this example shows, things don't always go as planned. This health professional interpreted the patient's request for information as distrust in his professional competence. His angry answer provoked an angry response from the patient, and the communication between the two broke down. The health professional began by intending to implement his treatment plan in a straightforward fashion. He understood how to treat the patient's disease, but he failed to understand the interpersonal behavior occurring between himself and his patient. His patient's behavior (making a request for information) affected his own behavior (he became angry), and his angry response affected the patient's behavior in turn (the patient got angry). What you do affects others; what others do affects you. If you are not aware of the basic principles of interpersonal behavior, things can get "out of hand" during patient interviews and interfere with your quality of care just as they did with the health professional in our example. The purpose of this chapter is to help you develop some basic skills in understanding interpersonal behavior.

B.   FOUR MODELS OF INTERPERSONAL BEHAVIOR

A model is a representation of reality. A map, for instance, is a model of the terrain it represents. Models condense certain aspects of reality to their most important features. A builder's blueprints for a house don't look like the finished product, but they represent the patterns to which the builder's materials must conform in order to build the house. A model of interpersonal behavior is a representation of certain important behaviors that occur in an interpersonal situation, such as a patient interview. The model directs your attention to those features of interpersonal behavior that the model-builder thinks you should know.

Four models of interpersonal behavior are listed below.

1.   COMMUNICATIONS MODEL
2.   TRANSACTIONAL ANALYSIS MODEL
3.   HUMAN NEEDS MODEL
4.   VALUES MODEL

Each model represents a different way of describing interpersonal behavior. There are many models of interpersonal behavior, but these four have been chosen because they are the most useful in understanding health care situations.

1.   Communications Model of Interpersonal Behavior

Communication is the process by which information is exchanged between two or more persons. The communication process involves five steps:

Step 1: Message Formation.   The message is formed in the mind of the sender.

Step 2: Message Encoding.   The sender translates (ENCODES) his idea (message) into a form that can be transmitted to the receiver. That is, the sender decides how to send his message in spoken or written words, or using body language (e.g., the extended hand that communicates the wish to greet another person).

Step 3: Message Transmission.   The sender transmits his message. For example, he mails a letter or he extends his hand.

Step 4: Message Reception.   The receiver perceives the message. He hears the speaker's words, or he sees the letter or the extended hand.

Step 5: Message Decoding.   The receiver translates (DECODES) what he has seen or heard to determine the meaning of the sender's message. (For example, "His hand is extended toward me. He's greeting me.")

When communication is successful, the message DECODED by the receiver is identical to the message formed and ENCODED by the sender. That is, if you are the receiver, you get the message the sender intended for you.

Now what has all this to do with health professionals? The diagram below (Figure 2.1) shows an example of a successful communication exchange between a health professional and a patient. Each wants to send the other a specific and important message, and each communicator does so successfully. The message received is virtually identical to the message formed in the mind of the sender and the message sent.

The formula for effective interpersonal communication is:

Message Formed = Message Sent = Message Received

This is an example of communication at its best, and if all communication between health professionals and patients were this good, we would have little need for a communications model of interpersonal behavior. Unfortunately, in many cases the communication between health professionals and patients breaks down. Frequently, the message received is not the same as the message that was sent or intended to be sent. When mis-

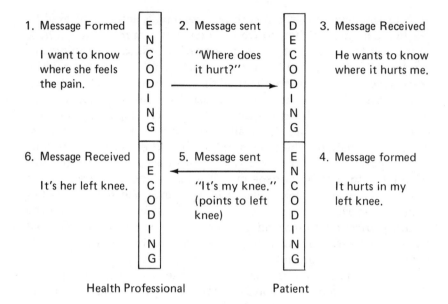

1. Message Formed

I want to know
where she feels
the pain.

ENCODING

2. Message sent

"Where does
it hurt?"

DECODING

3. Message Received

He wants to know
where it hurts me.

6. Message Received

It's her left knee.

DECODING

5. Message sent

"It's my knee."
(points to left
knee)

ENCODING

4. Message formed

It hurts in my
left knee.

Health Professional   Patient

FIGURE 2.1. Example of a Successful Communication Exchange

communication occurs, the health professional and the patient can encounter serious difficulty.

The gap between the message that is meant to be sent, the message that is actually sent, and the message that is received is called THE INTERPERSONAL GAP. It is a major source of misunderstanding between health professionals and patients. The two main types of INTERPERSONAL GAPS are described here.

ERROR IN THE TRANSMISSION OF A MESSAGE

Health Professional's Intended Message	Message Sent By Health Professional	Message Received By Patient	Patient's Reaction
(Thinks: I'm pleased to see Mrs. Smith.)	"Hello, Mrs. Smith. I'm pleased to see you." (Voice tone is cold, facial expression is impassive, there is no eye contact with patient.)	"I'm not really pleased to see you."	(Thinks: This is the last time I'll come to her for help.)

In this example, the health professional is actually pleased to see her patient, but her nonverbal behavior communicates a lack of interest to the patient. When a person's words say one thing and her "body language" says another, most people will interpret the body language as communicating the real message. Research has shown that the "real message" is usually conveyed nonverbally (e.g. through facial expression, other body language, or voice tone). In this example, the health professional may actually have disliked the patient; she may have acted cold because she thought it was part of her role as a health professional not to act too friendly with patients; or she may just have been unaware that her nonverbal behavior lacked warmth. Whatever the reason for her cold nonverbal behavior, the result is the same: the message the health professional *intended* to send to the patient is not received by the patient. This health professional makes an ENCODING error and fails to transmit her intended message clearly.

Three main ways of transmitting a message to another person are through speech (what you say), voice tone (how you say it), and body language (your facial and other body gestures).

When talking to a patient, you are invariably communicating through all three of these COMMUNICATION CHANNELS at the same time. If your message is the same in all three channels —

Speech: "I'm pleased to see you."

Voice tone: Your voice sounds warm.

Body language: You maintain frequent eye contact and smile.

— then your voice tone and body language will reinforce the message you have put into words. This is an example of CONGRUENT COMMUNICATION. If your nonverbal behavior detracts from your verbal message —

Speech: "I'm pleased to see you."

Voice tone: Your voice sounds cold.

Body language: You avoid eye contact with your patient.

— then your patient may get a message different from the one you intended. This is an example of an INCONGRUENT COMMUNICATION.

In the following example, the patient has requested information about his medication, but the health professional has misinterpreted the request as a challenge to his competence. The message the patient intended to send was sent correctly. The breakdown in communication occured at the receiving end where the health professional made a DECODING error and interpreted the patient's message incorrectly.

ERROR IN THE RECEPTION OF A MESSAGE

Patient's Intended Message	Message Sent By Patient	Message Received By Health Professional	Health Professional's Reaction
(Thinks: What are these pills for?)	"What are these pills for?"	I don't trust you.	(Thinks: How dare he treat me like this.)

In summary, the two main types of communication errors are ENCODING errors and DECODING errors. Figure 2.2 shows the point at which each error occurs in the communication process.

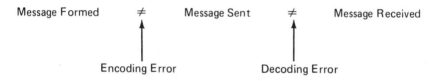

FIGURE 2.2. Errors in the Communication Process

Frequently, one or both types of communication errors will occur at the same time. The result can be a real communication mix-up.

Example

Several years ago in Hamilton, Ontario, there was a general transit strike, and no buses were running. A teenage patient who had walked some distance to get to the medical center had the following conversation with a health professional.

Health professional: "What brought you here today?"
Patient: "My feet."

The patient meant that he had walked to the medical center. The health professional, however, thought that the patient had come to the center because of a "foot problem" and proceeded to question the puzzled teenager about his feet for half an hour.

The communication errors that occurred in this example are shown in the following diagram (Figure 2.3):

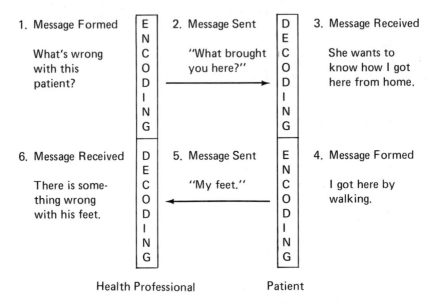

Health Professional   Patient

FIGURE 2.3. Communication Errors

In this communication sequence, the patient makes a DE-CODING error at step 3 when he misinterprets a standard inquiry. A second DECODING error occurs at step 6 when the health professional misinterprets the patient's correctly sent message. At this point the health professional and the patient are like two TV sets facing each other but tuned to different channels. Because this health professional was not sensitive to the possibility of communication errors, a serious INTERPERSONAL GAP resulted between her and the patient. If this type of communication error had occurred with a patient who had a more serious medical emergency, the consequences would have been more serious for both the patient and the health professional.

Exercise 4:   Identifying Interpersonal Gaps

Purpose: To identify INTERPERSONAL GAPS caused by communication errors that have occurred in your interactions with others.

Instructions: (a) In the spaces provided below, identify examples of ENCODING and DECODING errors that have occurred between yourself and others.

(b) Diagram your INTERPERSONAL GAP using the figure provided.

(c) Choose a partner and share your examples of INTERPERSONAL GAPS with him.

1. Briefly describe an incident in which you or another person made an *ENCODING* error. What negative consequences resulted, if any?

_____

_____

_____

_____

_____

Use the figure below (Figure 2.4) to diagram the communication process that occurred.

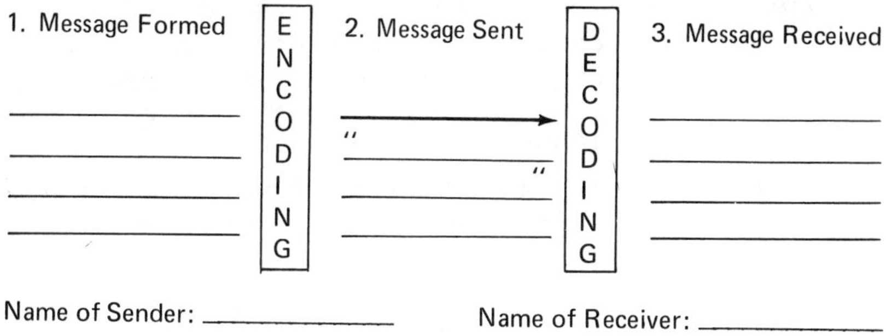

1. Message Formed | E N C O D I N G | 2. Message Sent | D E C O D I N G | 3. Message Received

Name of Sender: _____   Name of Receiver: _____

FIGURE 2.4.

2. Briefly describe an incident in which you or another person made a *DECODING* error. What negative consequences resulted, if any?

_____

_____

_____

_____

_____

Use the figure below (Figure 2.5) to diagram the communication process that occurred.

1. Message Formed   E   2. Message Sent   D   3. Message Received
                     N   E
                     C   C
_____   O   _____   O   _____
                     D   ''   D
_____   I   _____ '' I   _____
                     N   _____   N
_____   G   G   _____

_____   _____   _____

Name of Sender: _____   Name of Receiver: _____

FIGURE 2.5.

Exercise 5:   Understanding Decoding Errors

Purpose: To develop an appreciation for the ease with which DECODING communication errors can occur.

Instructions: 1(a)   Each member of the class should, on his own, examine the figure shown below and count up the number of triangles (any shape of triangle) in this figure. (Time: 10 minutes)

(b)   The group leader should next write down on the chalkboard each member's answer.

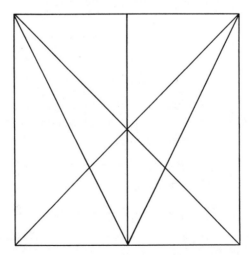

FIGURE 2.6.

Questions for Discussion

- Was there close agreement among the group members as to the number of triangles in the figure? If not, why not?
- What does this exercise demonstrate about problems in communication and in perception of another person's behavior?

2(a) Imagine that you are involved in the following situation. You are a health professional working at a local health clinic. You have a 2:30 p.m. appointment with a new patient. At 2 p.m. the secretary for the clinic calls and says, "Your 2:30 appointment — Mrs. Jones — just called and said she wouldn't be coming."

Write down as many alternative reasons as you can think of to explain why your patient didn't show up.

Alternative Explanations

1. _____
2. _____
3. _____
4. _____
5. _____
6. _____
7. _____
8. _____
9. _____
10. _____

(b) Circle the number of the alternative explanation that you think would most likely be true.

(c) Put an 'X' beside the alternative explanation that would upset you most if it were the true explanation.

Questions for Discussion

- How many alternative explanations were group members able to list?

- Did group members agree as to what sort of explanation was most likely to be true? (You may want to list these on a chalkboard to facilitate discussion.)
- What type of alternative explanation was most likely to upset group members?
- How is the principle of DECODING illustrated in this exercise?
- Have any group members actually experienced a situation like this? If so, what conclusions did they make about their patient's failure to show up?

Exercise 6:   One-Way and Two-Way Communication

Purpose: To understand the role of FEEDBACK in communication.

Instructions: 1. Before class, the group leader should prepare two drawings, each on blank, regular size (8½" x 11") paper. The first drawing should consist of *eight* rectangles (each one 1" x 2½") arranged in any pattern, but with each rectangle touching at least one other rectangle. For example, as in Figure 2.7:

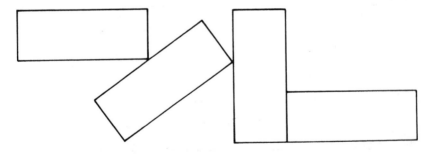

FIGURE 2.7.

The second drawing should also consist of eight rectangles, each touching another but arranged differently from the rectangles in the first drawing. These drawings should not be shown to the class prior to the exercise.

2. *Demonstration of one-way communication*
Each class member is given a blank 8½" x 11" piece of paper. The group leader, holding his

first drawing so that the rest of the group cannot see it, should describe slowly and in detail where each rectangle is on the page and how each is connected to the others. During the leader's description of his drawing, each class member should try to copy on his paper what he thinks the leader's drawing looks like. During this portion of the exercise, the class members are not allowed to ask the leader any questions or to talk to each other. After the leader has finished describing his drawing, he should hold it up so that the class can check their drawings. Each group member should write down the number of rectangles he copied down in the right spot.

3. *Demonstration of two-way communication*
Each class member is given a second blank sheet of paper. The group leader, holding his second drawing so that the class cannot see it, should describe it. This time, however, the class members can interrupt the leader at any time and ask questions about where each rectangle is. After about ten minutes, the leader should hold up his drawing so that the class can check the accuracy of their drawing and count up the number of rectangles correctly placed.

Questions for Discussion

- Which type of communication (one-way or two-way) was most effective in producing accurate reproductions of the leader's drawing? The leader can use the following headings to summarize scores on a chalkboard:

Type of Communication

	One Way	Two Way
Number of Rectangles Accurately Placed		

- Which type of communication took the shortest time?
- Do other health professionals you know mainly use one-way or two-way communication with their patients? What

are some negative consequences that might result when a health professional uses only one-way communication with patients?

2.   Transactional Analysis Model of Interpersonal Behavior

Transactional Analysis is the study of the communication or TRANSACTIONS that take place between people and of the sometimes unconscious and destructive ways ("games") that people relate to each other. This approach to personality was developed by Eric Berne, a psychiatrist who made Transactional Analysis (TA for short) a popular theory through his book, *Games People Play.*

Overview of Berne's Theory.   The cornerstone of Berne's theory is that each person's personality is made up of three distinct parts called EGO STATES. An ego state is a consistent pattern of feeling, experiencing, and behaving. The three ego states that make up your personality are: the Parent ego state (PARENT); the Adult ego state (ADULT), and the Child ego state (CHILD). The ego states are diagrammed as shown below in Figure 2.8:

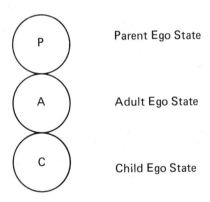

FIGURE 2.8. Your personality is made up of ego states

Berne first became aware of ego states while treating a thirty-five-year-old lawyer who told Berne, "I'm not really a lawyer. I'm just a little boy." What the lawyer meant was that during treatment he felt and acted like he was a child. In the outside world, he was a competent lawyer. Berne referred to these two "selves" as "the CHILD" (the part of the lawyer's self that felt insecure and like a little kid) and "the ADULT" (the part of the lawyer's self that dealt with his work in a rational, competent manner). Berne later discovered a third "self," "the PARENT," which is the part of one's personality that acts parental (stern, authoritarian, prejudiced, or nurturing).

Have you ever had someone yell at you and then found yourself feeling intimidated and scared, just like when you were a little kid and the school bully shouted at you? Did you ever have to speak in front of a large group and found yourself feeling anxious just like the first time you had to speak in front of the class in grade school? If you did, then you were experiencing your Child ego state.

Have you ever had someone yell at you, but you calmly said to them, "What's the matter?" and tried to analyze what was wrong? Have you ever become so absorbed while studying a problem (in school or work) that you forgot there were other people around you? Did you ever try to figure out how a piece of equipment works, or why someone acts the way he or she does? If you did, then you were experiencing your Adult ego state.

Have you ever ordered someone around just the way your parents might have once ordered you to do something, "Stop that at once!", "Don't do that!", "Come here this minute!", "Do it now!"? Have you ever comforted someone when he was upset and put your arm around him and said (just the way you once saw your mother or father do), "There now, don't worry, it's going to be all right."? Have you ever scolded someone, just the way your mother or father might have once scolded you, "How dare you speak to me like that!", "You *never* listen", "Can't you do anything right?" If you did, you were experiencing your Parent ego state.

According to Berne, your personality is made up of these three ego states: PARENT, ADULT, and CHILD. It's as though you have three "people" inside you: the Parent-you, which incorporates all the attitudes and behavior you were *taught* (directly or indirectly) by your parents; the Child-you, which contains all the *feelings* you had as a child; and the Adult-you, which deals with reality in a logical, *rational*, computer-like manner. These three ego states are distinct, each having a consistent pattern of feeling, experiencing, and behaving.

The Parent and Child ego states are essentially made up of feelings, attitudes, and behaviors recorded in your brain—much like on a high quality videotape recorder—up to the age of about five or six. When you are confronted with situations in your adult life that are *similar* to the situations that produced your earliest Parent or Child "recordings," you may re-experience those early feelings and attitudes again, almost in flashback fashion. When someone shouts at you, you may want to keep cool, but your CHILD "tapes" may play nevertheless, and you feel the same fear and anxiety you once felt as a child when confronted with an angry parent or the school bully.

The Parent and the Child ego states are remnants from the past, stored up in your brain as high quality recordings that can be replayed in the future. Evidence for this comes from the work of the noted neurologist William Penfield who showed that when he stimulated different parts of a patient's brain electrically, the patient would "see" and "hear" things that had happened to him or her in the past. Not only would the patient remember a specific childhood event such as walking in his father's apple orchard, he would *experience* the same feelings he felt on that day, when as a child, he walked through the orchard and felt especially happy. The significance of Penfield's research is that it shows that everything that happened to you is stored up in your brain—not only the memory of what happened, but also the emotions that went along with the specific experience. Under the right conditions, your Child and Parent tapes will "play" and you will not only remember how you once felt critical or sad, you will actually re-experience the emotions you felt and the beliefs you had in the original situation.

SUMMARY

The Parent Ego State.   (See Figure 2.9.) This is like a videotape recording of all the nurturing, critical, and prejudicial attitudes, behaviors, and experiences learned from other people, especially parents and teachers. For example, the person who had very authoritarian parents may learn from them similar authoritarian attitudes and behavior. Under the right conditions, he will act in a critical or prejudicial manner, just as he once saw his parents do. When this occurs, we say that he is in his Parent ego state. There are two parts to the Parent Ego State: the CRITICAL PARENT and the NURTURING PARENT. When you are authoritarian and "bossy," that is your CRITICAL PARENT. When you are protective of, and nurturing toward, others, that is your NURTURING PARENT. When you are in your Parent Ego State you are expressing attitudes, feelings, and behaviors you have *uncritically* learned from other persons.

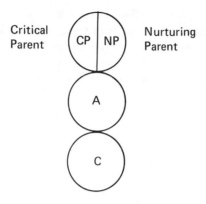

FIGURE 2.9. The Parent Ego State

The Adult Ego State.   (See Figure 2.10.) This is the part of the personality that is like a computer: it gathers and processes information about the world and is objective, emotionless, and intelligent in its approach to problem solving. Even young children have an Adult ego state. The ADULT is the reality-oriented part of the personality. Unlike the Parent ego state, which records and "replays" the attitudes and behaviors of others, the ADULT analyzes the information it gathers and checks it out—reality tests it—before computing a course of action. When you solve a problem, estimate probabilities, or think about alternatives, you are in your Adult ego state.

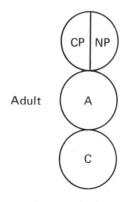

FIGURE 2.10. The Adult Ego State

The Child Ego State.   (See Figure 2.11.) This contains all the feelings, attitudes, and behaviors you had as a young child. Your childhood experiences are stored in the Child Ego State as on a videotape recorder and can be replayed so that you recall or re-experience the feelings and beliefs you had as a child.

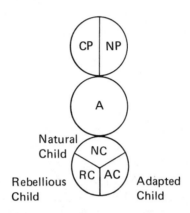

FIGURE 2.11. The Child Ego State

When you are feeling happy and spontaneous, that is your NATURAL CHILD—the you as you were, uninhibited by the sanctions of adults.

The ADAPTED CHILD is the part of the Child Ego State that has been modified by parents and the social environment. This is the part of the CHILD that adapts its natural inclinations (the spontaneous impulses in the NATURAL CHILD) to meet parental and social demands. Common ADAPTED CHILD behaviors are: complying, acting "good," crying, being upset, withdrawing, being depressed. All of these behaviors represent different child reactions to parental demands—demands that force the child to adapt his behavior in some way from the NATURAL CHILD behavior that would be present if there were no parental demands made.

The REBELLIOUS CHILD is actually a part of the ADAPTED CHILD and represents counterdependent, rebellious, resistant behavior, usually learned in response to excessive parental demands.

The CHILD is above all the feeling part of the personality. In it reside feelings of happiness, joy, sadness, depression, anxiety, anger, rebellion. When you feel these emotions, you are experiencing in your CHILD ego state.

The ego states may be compared in the following examples, which show patients and health professionals interacting with different ego states.

Situation 1:   Adult–Adult Transaction

Patient: What exactly is wrong with me?

Health professional: You have a slight viral infection, but it's not serious.

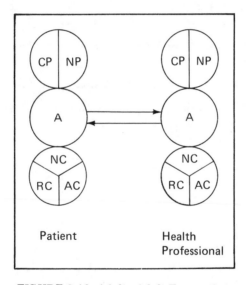

FIGURE 2.12. Adult -Adult Transaction

Situation 2:   Critical Parent–Critical Parent Transaction

Health professional #1:   Some patients are so irresponsible nowadays.

Health professional #2:   The way they don't take their pills— there ought to be a law!

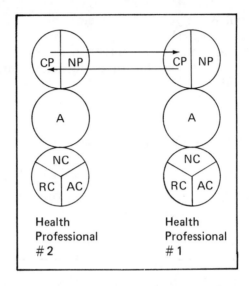

FIGURE 2.13. Critical Parent–Critical Parent Transaction

Situation 3:   Natural Child–Natural Child Transaction

Female patient #1:   Boy, did you see that handsome intern?
Female patient #2:   Yeah, what a doll!

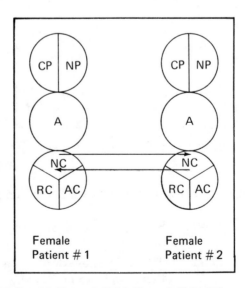

FIGURE 2.14. Natural Child–Natural Child Transaction

Situation 4:   Natural Child–Natural Child Transaction

Health professional #3:   Wow, that film on cardiovascular disease was great!

Health professional #4:   Yeah, fantastic!

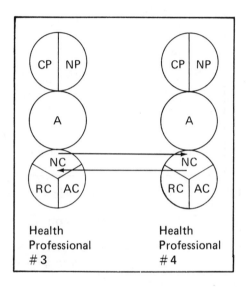

FIGURE 2.15. Natural Child–Natural Child Transaction

Situation 5:   Critical Parent–Adapted Child Transaction

Health professional supervisor: Good grief, that patient interview you just conducted was one of the worst I've ever seen.

Health professional student: I'm sorry . . . . I didn't mean to blow it. I'm really sorry.

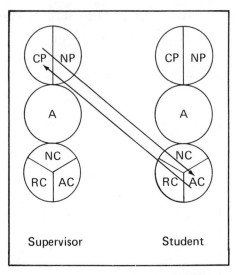

FIGURE 2.16. Critical Parent–Adapted Child Transaction

Situation 6:   Critical Parent–Rebellious Child Transaction

Health professional: Now see here young lady, if you want to get well, you're going to have to take your medicine every day.

Patient (age 12):   No! You can't make me take those stupid pills.

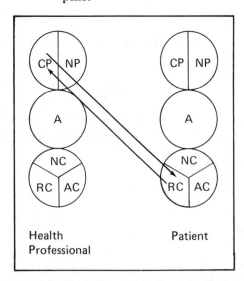

FIGURE 2.17. Critical Parent–Rebellious Child Transaction

The six examples shown are all complementary transactions, that is transactions where the arrows in the ego state diagrams are parallel. When a transaction between two people is complementary ("parallel arrows"), the conversation flows smoothly. If the arrows in the ego state diagram cross, communication breaks down. An example of such a CROSSED TRANSACTION was shown earlier in the chapter:

Example of a Crossed Transaction

Health professional: Take these pills for a week and then come back and see me.

Patient: What are these pills for? Could you tell me more about what they're supposed to do and any side effects they might have?

Health professional: (Getting angry): Look, if you don't trust me, then perhaps you should go see another health professional.

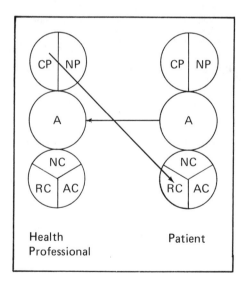

FIGURE 2.18. Crossed Transaction

Whether or not you accept Berne's theory about ego states, ego state diagrams are a convenient way of diagramming the different ways health professionals and patients interact with each other.

Exercise 7:   Analyzing Transactions Between Ego States

Purpose: To develop skills in identifying ego states. To develop skills in diagramming transactions between ego states.

Instructions: In each of the examples shown, diagram the transactions between the ego states of the persons in the example.

Situation 1

Patient: I feel so sick. I hurt so bad. What's happening to me? (Starts to cry.)

Health professional: There now . . . there now . . . don't worry. We'll look after you.

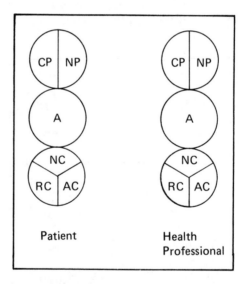

FIGURE 2.19. Situation #1

Situation 2

Health professional: Would you please roll up your sleeve so I can take a blood sample?

Patient: Certainly.

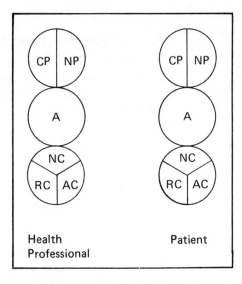

FIGURE 2.20. Situation #2

Situation 3

Health professional: I've had enough of this nonsense. You stay in that bed or else.

Patient, age 10:   I don't have to do what you tell me.

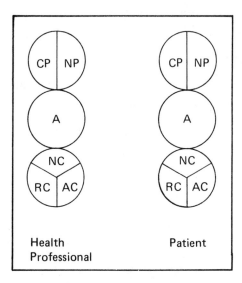

FIGURE 2.21. Situation #3

Situation 4

Patient: These exercises you've been having me do—
what exactly are they for?

Health professional: Now we're not going to go all over that
again are we? You just do what I told you,
and you'll feel a lot better.

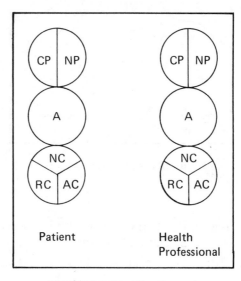

FIGURE 2.22. Situation #4

Situation 5

Health professional #1:   Say, I really like working with you.

Health professional #2:   I like you, too!

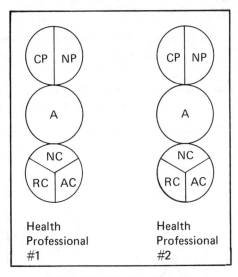

FIGURE 2.23. Situation #5

Situation 6

Patient: You seem rather young to be working here. I want someone *experienced.*

Health professional student: Uh . . . oh . . . ah . . . yes sir. I'll get someone else.

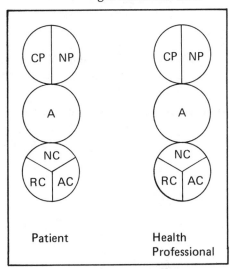

FIGURE 2.24. Situation #6

Situation 7

Patient: You seem rather young to be working here. I want someone *experienced*.

Health professional student: Look, if you don't like the service, mister, you can go somewhere else.

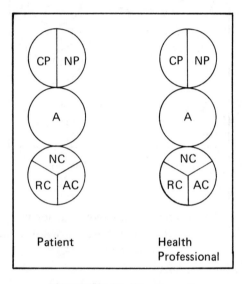

FIGURE 2.25. Situation #7

Situation 8

Patient: You seem rather young to be working here. I want someone *experienced*.

Health professional student: I may be young, but that doesn't mean I'm not experienced. Now, how can I help you?

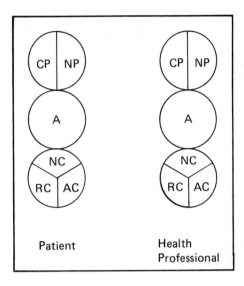

FIGURE 2.26. Situation #8

Exercise 8:   The Ego State Inventory

Purpose: To identify the ego states through which you express your personality. To explore the implications of different ego states for health professionals.

Instructions: 1. Each group member should complete and score the EGO STATE INVENTORY shown below.

Instructions for EGO STATE INVENTORY: Show the extent to which you feel you display each of the following characteristics by placing a check (✓) mark in the appropriate column to the right.

Are You Someone Who	A Great Deal	Moder- ately	Mildly	Not At All
1. Comforts others.				
2. Does not react emotionally.				
3. Uses expressions like "Wow!", "Gosh!", "Golly!", "Gee!".				
4. Ignores the leader.				

Are You Someone Who	A Great Deal	Moder- ately	Mildly	Not At All
5. Disapproves of the way others behave.				
6. Shows sympathy for others.				
7. Always disagrees.				
8. Is spontaneous with his (her) feelings.				
9. Acts shy.				
10. Likes to talk about "intellec- tual" things: eg. politics, economics, current affairs.				
11. Tries to please others.				
12. Stands up for others.				
13. Is good at solving problems.				
14. Is mean to others.				
15. Always conforms to the rules.				
16. Argues with others.				
17. Laughs and jokes a lot.				
18. Gets upset easily.				
19. Is critical of others.				
20. Protects the weak.				
21. Is a clear thinker.				
22. Often acts like a "big" kid.				
23. Tells others what they should, or ought, to do.				

Are You Someone Who	A Great Deal	Moderately	Mildly	Not At All
24. Acts helpless.				
25. Trusts others.				
26. Is stubborn.				
27. Often says or does silly things.				
28. Acts superior to others.				
29. Looks at the facts realistically.				
30. Is excessively polite.				
31. Likes to help others with their problems.				
32. Acts nervous.				
33. Withholds his (her) cooperation passively.				
34. Is able to see both sides of the situation.				
35. Is fun to be with.				
36. Will not do what he (she) is told.				
37. Tries to dominate others.				
38. Is very rational.				
36. Is a good person to talk to about one's personal problems.				
40. Refuses to do assigned work.				

Are You Someone Who	A Great Deal	Moder- ately	Mildly	Not At All
41. Is considerate of other people's feelings.				
42. Points out others' mistakes to them.				

SCORING KEY FOR EGO STATE INVENTORY

Instructions: 1. For each characteristic you have checked in the inventory, circle the number (score) in the corresponding space shown on this scoring key (eg., for characteristic #1, "comforts others" if you checked "A GREAT DEAL," then circle 3 for Q.1 on this sheet). 2. Total the scores for each Ego State and transfer these scores to the Results Sheet. For example, for the Ego State CP (Critical Parent) add together the scores for questions 5, 14, 19, 23, 28, 37 and 42.

Q.	A Great Deal	Moderately	Mildly	Not At All	Ego State
1	3	2	1	0	NP
2	3	2	1	0	A
3	3	2	1	0	NC
4	3	2	1	0	RC
5	3	2	1	0	CP
6	3	2	1	0	NP
7	3	2	1	0	RC
8	3	2	1	0	NC
9	3	2	1	0	AC

Q.	A Great Deal	Moderately	Mildly	Not At All	Ego State
10	3	2	1	0	A
11	3	2	1	0	AC
12	3	2	1	0	NP
13	3	2	1	0	A
14	3	2	1	0	CP
15	3	2	1	0	AC
16	3	2	1	0	RC
17	3	2	1	0	NC
18	3	2	1	0	AC
19	3	2	1	0	CP
20	3	2	1	0	NP
21	3	2	1	0	A
22	3	2	1	0	NC
23	3	2	1	0	CP
24	3	2	1	0	AC
25	3	2	1	0	NC
26	3	2	1	0	RC
27	3	2	1	0	NC
28	3	2	1	0	CP
29	3	2	1	0	A
30	3	2	1	0	AC

Q.	A Great Deal	Moderately	Mildly	Not At All	Ego State
31	3	2	1	0	NP
32	3	2	1	0	AC
33	3	2	1	0	RC
34	3	2	1	0	A
35	3	2	1	0	NC
36	3	2	1	0	RC
37	3	2	1	0	CP
38	3	2	1	0	A
39	3	2	1	0	NP
40	3	2	1	0	RC
41	3	2	1	0	NP
42	3	2	1	0	CP

RESULTS SHEET FOR EGO STATE INVENTORY

Instructions: 1. After transferring your scores from the SCOR-
ING   SHEET   to the spaces   provided   under the
column   "Score,"   calculate   percentage   scores.
(For example, if your Critical Parent score is 4/21,
your percentage score is 4/21 $\times$ 100 = 19%.)

Ego State Number	Ego State	Score	%
1	Critical Parent (CP)	——— / 21	———
2	Nurturing Parent (NP)	——— / 21	———
3	Adult (A)	——— / 21	———
4	Adapted Child (AC)	——— / 21	———

Ego State Number	Ego State	Score	%
5	Rebellious Child (RC)	____	____
		21	
6	Natural Child (NC)	____	____
		21	
* * * * * *	* * * * * * *	* *	* * * *
7	Total Parent (add 1 + 2)	____	____
		42	
8	Total Adult (3)	____	____
		21	
9	Total Child (add 4 + 5 + 6)	____	____
		63	
10	Anger-related Ego States (add 1 + 5)	____	____
		42	
11	Loving-related Ego States (add 2 + 6)	____	____
		42 .	

2. *Discussion procedure:* After each group member has completed his EGO STATE INVENTORY, the group leader can write the ego states (CP, NP, A, AC, RC, NC) on a chalkboard and then place a check in the columns under the two ego states he scored highest on for his self-rating. The rest of the group can then be invited to come up and do the same with their scores. The total number of check marks under each ego state can be totalled, and the two highest totals (indicating the two dominant ego states for the group as a whole) circled.

Questions for Discussion

- What was your strongest ego state? Weakest ego state?
- What were the strongest and weakest ego states for the entire group?
- What are the advantages and the disadvantages for health professionals of the dominant ego states identified?

Exercise 9:   Analyzing Your Transactions with Other People

Purpose: To develop skill in identifying transactions between your ego states and the ego states of other people with whom you interact.

Instructions: 1(a)   Briefly describe an enjoyable conversation you recently had with another person (a patient, health professional, friend, etc.). What did you say and do? What did the other person say and do?

What you said/did:

_____

_____

What the other person said/did:

_____

_____

(b)   Use the ego state diagram below (Figure 2.27) to summarize the transactions that occurred between you and the other person.

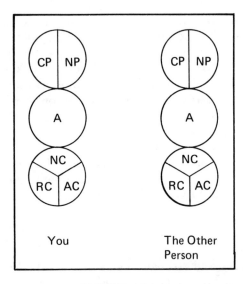

FIGURE 2.27.

2(a)   Briefly describe an *unpleasant* conversation you recently had with another person (a patient, health professional, friend, etc.). What did you say and do? What did the other person say and do?

What you said/did:

_____

_____

What the other person said/did:

_____

_____

(b) Use the ego state diagram below (Figure 2.28) to summarize the transactions that occurred between you and the other person.

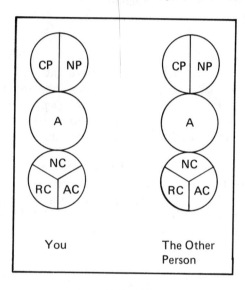

FIGURE 2.28.

3. Group Discussion: The group can be divided into pairs. Each pair can spend 10 minutes sharing their incidents and ego state diagrams.

Questions for Discussion

- What ego states were most frequently involved in an enjoyable conversation?
- What ego states were most frequently involved in an unpleasant conversation?

3.   Human Needs Model of
Interpersonal Behavior

The human needs model of interpersonal behavior emphasizes that all humans have the same basic needs and that these needs are what motivates a person's behavior. A need is an urge experienced by a person to achieve a goal that will satisfy the urge. For example, if you feel hungry (need) you may buy and eat a hamburger (goal) to satisfy your hunger. Hunger is one of the most basic of human needs. When your hunger need is activated it has a powerful, directing effect on your behavior.

Example

Mary is a health professional working in a large metropolitan hospital. One morning she is late for work and skips breakfast. At 11 a.m. during her third patient interview, she starts to feel hunger pangs and a little weak. The patient is talking about something important, but Mary finds it difficult to pay attention.

As this example shows, when your hunger need is not satisfied, it can interfere with your patient interviews.

The psychologist Abraham Maslow has described five basic categories of needs: PHYSIOLOGICAL NEEDS (the need to eat, sleep, breathe, eliminate, avoid pain, etc.), SAFETY NEEDS (the need to be free from fear of physical harm), BELONGING NEEDS (the need to be loved, to belong), ESTEEM NEEDS (the need to feel good about yourself through achievement, independence; the positive valuation of yourself by yourself and others), and SELF-ACTUALIZATION (the need to creatively fulfill your potential).

These needs can be arranged in a pyramid (see Figure 2.29) with the most basic needs, those requiring immediate—or near-immediate—satisfaction to maintain life (i.e., PHYSIOLOGICAL NEEDS) at the bottom. The needs at the top of the pyramid are important, but not as critical as those lower down. For example, a patient who is in intense pain from a knee injury (his PHYSIOLOGICAL NEED to be free from pain is unsatisfied) is unlikely to be too concerned at that moment with whether or not he is successful at his job (ESTEEM NEED level). According to Maslow, as you satisfy each lower need level to an adequate degree, you will become increasingly concerned with satisfying your next, or higher, need level. As each need level becomes satisfied, you become concerned with a different set of goal-seeking behaviors directed at your higher need levels. In this sense, some needs are

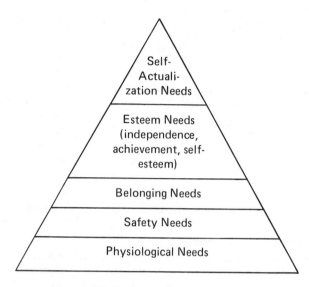

FIGURE 2.29. Maslow's Pyramid of Needs

more basic than others. The lower a need is in the pyramid, the more driving a force it will tend to have on a person's behavior in comparison with the "higher" needs.

This model of human needs can be used to explain interpersonal behavior between patients and health professionals. This is illustrated by the following example taken from earlier in the chapter:

EXAMPLE OF DIFFERENT NEEDS IN AN INTERVIEW

Dialogue	*Dominant Need Present*
Health professional: "Take these pills for a week and then come back and see me."	No dominant need.
Patient: "What are these pills for? Could you tell me more about what they're supposed to do and any side effects they might have?"	*SAFETY NEED.* This patient works at a job where he operates heavy equipment. The presence of any side effects in his medication—such as drowsiness—could result in a fatal accident.
Health professional: (Getting angry) "Look, if you don't trust me, then perhaps you should go see another health professional."	*ESTEEM.* The health professional interprets the patient's request for information as an attack on his competence. The health professional feels put-down; his esteem

Dialogue	*Dominant Need Present*
	is at stake. He tries to satisfy his esteem need by "fighting back."
Patient: (Getting angry) "Look, if you don't know how to answer a simple question, maybe you shouldn't be practicing health care."	*ESTEEM.* The patient feels put-down by the health professional's remark. The patient feels discounted, devalued by the health professional, and tries to protect his esteem by "fighting back" as well.

In this example, if the health professional had perceived that the patient's question about medication was motivated by a SAFETY NEED, he would have responded with information and understanding, rather than with defensiveness and aggression. Understanding the different needs that motivate patients can help make a health professional more effective. Perhaps the key thing to remember is: Just because patients come to see a health professional primarily for their physiological needs doesn't mean that their other needs can be ignored.

Exercise 10:   Identifying Types of Human Needs

Purpose: To develop your skills in identifying the different kinds of human needs described by Maslow.

Instructions: Read each statement below and write in the space provided the need that you feel is most likely the dominant need felt by the person speaking. The needs you can choose are listed below.

Needs

PHYSIOLOGICAL
SAFETY
BELONGING
ESTEEM
SELF-ACTUALIZATION

Situation 1

Patient to Health professional: "The pain in my back is killing me. You've got to give me something for it!"

Need present: _____

Situation 2

Patient A to Patient B: "It gets pretty lonely in the ward on the weekends. My daughter doesn't come by very often."

Need present: _____

Situation 3

Health professional A to Health professional B: "I feel really bored by this job. I mean, I do it well—everybody says so—but somehow, it's just not enough."

Need present: _____

Situation 4

Six-year-old patient to health professional: "No! No! I don't want my blood taken." (Starts to cry.)

Need present: _____

Situation 5

Patient in bed to health professional: "I called five times and nobody answered. Don't you people know how to treat patients with a little dignity?"

Need present: _____

Situation 6

Health professional B to Health professional C: "Boy did I make a mess out of my case presentation—it was a real disaster. I feel like a complete idiot."

Need present: _____

Situation 7

Patient to Health professional: "It's been a week since I had my surgery, and I still feel so weak. Is it possible I might die?"

Need present: _____

Situation 8

Mother of 3-year-old patient to Health professional: "Just one minute! What do you mean my baby needs a better diet? Are you saying I don't know how to be a good mother?"

Need present: _____

Exercise 11:   Analyzing Needs in Yourself and in Others

Purpose: To develop skills in analyzing how needs motivate your behavior and the behavior of others. To identify ways of showing others that you understand their needs.

Instructions: Each group member should answer questions 1 to 4 on his own.

Part I: Analyzing Your Own Needs

1(a) Briefly describe a time you felt really happy.

_____

_____

_____

(b) What need in you was being satisfied? _____

2(a) Briefly, describe a time you felt upset or dissatisfied.

_____

_____

_____

(b) What need in you was unsatisfied? _____

(c) What action did you take to satisfy your need? Were you successful in satisfying your need?

_____

_____

_____

Part II: Analyzing Needs in Others

3(a) Briefly describe an incident in which you noticed a patient or health professional who seemed really happy.

_____

_____

_____

(b) What need was this person satisfying? _____

4(a) Briefly describe an incident in which you noticed a patient or health professional who seemed really upset or dissatisfied.

_____

_____

_____

(b) What need in this person was unsatisfied?_____

(c) Describe one way this person could be helped to satisfy his or her need. (Try to think of something *you* could have said or done to be helpful.)

_____

_____

_____

Group debriefing: To debrief the exercise, the group can be divided into pairs. Each pair should spend about 10 minutes sharing responses to questions 1 and 2 (Part 1). To debrief questions 3 and 4 (Part II), each pair can join with another pair to form groups of 4 (class size permitting). Responses to part II can then be shared in this "larger" group setting.

Questions for Discussion

- What satisfied needs were most frequently selected as making group members happy?
- What needs, when unsatisfied, were most frequently selected as making group members dissatisfied?
- What satisfied needs were most frequently selected as making patients or health professionals happy?
- What unsatisfied needs were most frequently selected as making patients or health professionals dissatisfied?

- For what need(s) in others was it most difficult to think of a way to satisfy the need (see question 4c).
- Why is it important for health professionals to satisfy their own needs?

4. Values Model of Interpersonal Behavior

Values are the general activities, characteristics, or ways of being that you prize. A person's values are his standards for correct behavior. Your values are your preferences for a particular way of life.

A value, however, is not the same as an activity. The same activity can be used to express different values. For example, someone may play golf because he values:

1. LEISURE (he finds golf relaxing—it takes his mind off his difficult job as a health professional);
2. COMPETITION (he plays golf for the challenge, the thrill of competing with and beating his golf partners);
3. PHYSICAL FITNESS (he golfs to keep his weight down and his muscles fit); or
4. FRIENDSHIP (he golfs because it is an activity he can share with his friends—it is a mutual activity that brings them closer together).

Similarly, someone may choose to become a health professional because she values:

1. INDEPENDENCE (she expects to earn enough money so that she will never have to be dependent on others);
2. HELPING OTHERS (she wants to alleviate sickness and suffering in the world);
3. STATUS (she wants others to look up to her and respect her);
4. CREATIVITY (she sees being a health professional as a way of actualizing herself, of reaching her full potential as a person); or
5. DUTY (she wants to become a health professional because her parents expect it of her).

There are many more values than can be listed here that can motivate one to become a health professional. Values are more general than *specific* interests or activities. Typically, an interest or activity is the means through which a value is expressed.

Values are important because—like needs—they affect interpersonal behavior.

Example of Values

Dialogue	Value Present
Health professional: "Take these pills for a week, and then come back and see me."	*HELPING OTHERS.* The health professional instructs the patient in a way that the health professional believes will benefit the patient.
Patient: "What are these pills for? Could you tell me more about what they're supposed to do and any side effects they might have?	*INDEPENDENCE.* The patient values "standing up on his own two feet" and taking responsibility for looking after his health. He seeks the information from the health professional that will enable him to do this.
	EQUALITY. The patient sees the health professional as an equal. The patient views himself as a customer who has a right to complete information from the health professional who is there to serve him.
Health professional: (Getting angry) "Look, if you don't trust me, then perhaps you should go see another health professional."	*AUTHORITY.* The health professional believes that because he is the expert he has the authority to withhold or give information to patients. Competence is the basis for his authority and this authority should be respected. Patients who do not respect authority are "bad" patients.
Patient: (Getting angry) "Look, if you don't know how to answer a simple question, maybe you shouldn't be practicing health care."	*EQUALITY.* The patient feels he has a right to this information. He believes that health professionals who act "authoritarian" and treat him as unequal are "bad" health professionals.

This example nicely illustrates how two opposing values—Authority and Equality—can result in conflict between patients and health professionals.

Values are learned attitudes. Values are learned from our parents, teachers, and "significant others." Different people hold different values. Even people who hold similar values may rank-order them differently according to importance. When patients and health professionals hold different values, the potential for conflict or misunderstanding may become high. By understanding how your patients' values differ from your own, you will be able to communicate more effectively with your patients.

Exercise 12:   Values Clarification Exercise

Purpose: To develop an awareness of your own values. To develop an awareness of, and a respect for, the values that other people hold.

To develop skills in identifying the ways your values can help or hinder your work as a health professional.

Instructions:

Part I

1. Each group member on his own writes down what he feels to be his personal values in the space provided below. Identify as many values (up to 10) as you can. Next, beside each value you have identified, list one example of how you express your value in everyday life. (For example: If one of your values is leisure, you might express this value by going sailing on the weekends.) After you have listed your personal values and examples, circle the two values you consider most important in your life.

My Personal Values	*Examples of How I Express My Values*
a) _____	_____
b) _____	_____
c) _____	_____
d) _____	_____
e) _____	_____

f) _____   _____

g) _____   _____

h) _____   _____

i) _____   _____

j) _____   _____

2. Divide the group into groups of 5 or 6. Each group can debrief the exercise by having each group member, in turn, read out his list of values and examples to the group. How much information a group member shares should be up to that person. After a group member has shared his values (and pointed out his top two values), the rest of the group members should tell the "presenter" which of his values they liked best.

3. If there are two or more groups in the class, each group should next determine what values the group members hold in common. A spokesman for each group can read out the "group values," and the group leader can write these down on a chalkboard to facilitate discussion. The group leader, together with the class, should identify the 5 most commonly held values in the class. Each group member should write these 5 values into the table shown below.

The group members should return to their groups of 5 (or 6) and try to achieve *consensus* on what they feel is the *main* advantage and the *main* disadvantage of each value listed as it might affect a health professional's work. (For example: if one of the values is Privacy, an advantage might be that the health professional who holds this value will respect the rights and privacy of his patients. A possible disadvantage is that he might be reluctant to self-disclose personal information about himself in the group and this might hinder learning new behaviors.)

The Group's Main Values	Main Advantage	Main Disadvantage

a) _____   _____   _____

b) _____   _____   _____

The Group's Main Values	Main Advantage	Main Disadvantage
c) _____	_____	_____
d) _____	_____	_____
e) _____	_____	_____

4. The group leader can debrief the exercise by having the different groups report on what they saw as the main advantage and main disadvantage for the first value, then continue with the next value, etc.

Questions for Discussion

- What value was chosen most frequently by group members?
- Was there high agreement on the values selected—or a wide diversity of choices?
- What value seemed to have the greatest advantage? Greatest disadvantage?

Exercise 13:   Analyzing Interpersonal Behavior

Purpose: To develop skills in analyzing your interaction with others using the four models of interpersonal behavior: COMMUNICATIONS MODEL, TRANSACTIONAL ANALYSIS MODEL, HUMAN NEEDS MODEL, and VALUES MODEL.

Instructions:

1. Briefly describe a recent incident in which there was a breakdown in the communication between you and a patient or health professional. Describe what you said and did and what the other person said and did. How did you feel? How do you think the other person felt?

_____

_____

_____

_____

_____

_____

_____

2. Now analyze this incident using the communications, transactional analysis, human needs, and values models. You can
   use the diagrams and tables below to summarize what you
   feel were the essential features of the incident. One model
   may apply more than the others in analyzing your situation.
   Nevertheless, try and view the interpersonal situation from
   the viewpoint of all four models.

(a) *COMMUNICATIONS MODEL*

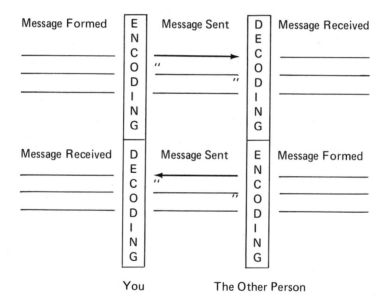

Check (✓) the type of communication error (INTERPERSON-
AL GAP) that occurred:

	Error made by	
	You	*The Other Person*
ENCODING error	_____	_____
DECODING error	_____	_____

(b) *TRANSACTIONAL ANALYSIS MODEL*

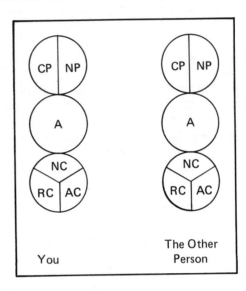

(c) *HUMAN NEEDS MODEL*

	You	*The Other Person*
Needs Present In:		

(d) *VALUES MODEL*

	You	*The Other Person*
Values Present In:		

3. From your current understanding of this incident, how would you have handled the incident differently (more effectively)?

_____

_____

_____

4. *Debriefing:* The leader can divide the group into pairs and have each group member share her analysis with her partner.

Questions for Discussion

- Which model of interpersonal behavior seems most useful for *describing* interpersonal behavior?
- Which model seems most useful for *explaining* interpersonal behavior? (N.B. description refers to what happens; explanation refers to *why* it happens.)
- What other models have group members found useful for describing and explaining interpersonal behavior?

SUMMARY

The four models of interpersonal behavior described in this chapter are different ways of looking at the same behavior. To use an analogy: a street scene may be photographed, filmed in color, videotaped in black and white, painted onto a canvas, described on a tape recorder, or described in print. All are different ways of describing the same street scene—with each method giving a different perspective. Similarly, the communications, transactional analysis, human needs, and values models of interpersonal behavior are complementary ways of describing and explaining interpersonal behavior. Each views interpersonal behavior from a slightly different perspective. The effective health professional is able to use all four models to make sense of his interaction with patients and to avoid any breakdowns in communication.

3

Developing Skills
for Coping with
Interpersonal Stress

A. WHAT IS INTERPERSONAL STRESS?

Interpersonal stress is tension you experience when you interact with another person who is behaving in a way you find unpleasant. For example, if a patient looks impatient and speaks to you in a sarcastic tone—you may find yourself tensing up, feeling nervous, and wishing you could be somewhere else. In this instance, the patient's angry behavior is a stressor for you—it makes you feel stressed in a negative way. This is summarized in Figure 3.1.

STRESSOR ⟶ STRESS

(Angry patient)   (Tense health professional)

FIGURE 3.1   Patient's angry behavior produces stress in the health professional

1. The Most Common Interpersonal Stressors

An INTERPERSONAL STRESSOR is a type of behavior exhibited by another person that has a negative impact on you. The ten most common stressors experienced by health professionals are:

1. Commands
2. Anger
3. Criticism
4. Unresponsiveness
5. Depression
6. Impulsivity
7. Affection
8. Making mistakes
9. Sexual content
10. Pain

COMMANDS are orders to do something. Although the person giving the command may be very calm, he will convey the attitude that he expects his command to be obeyed.

Example

Your supervisor comes up to you and says:

Supervisor: Go to ward C and take Miss Parker's blood pressure right away.

ANGER is strong displeasure, most commonly expressed by yelling, insults, tense facial muscles, a flushed face, a clenched fist, and other "fight" gestures.

Example

You arrive at clinic half an hour late for your patient's appointment. Your patient, Mr. Jones, is red-faced and pacing back and forth in the examination room. When he sees you, he walks up to you and shakes his finger in your face.

Mr. Jones: Now see here! My time is valuable, and I don't like being kept waiting by some arrogant health professional who thinks I've got nothing better to do than cool my heels in a waiting room. Hurry up!

CRITICISM is disapproval expressed by mildly negative comments, pointing out another's faults, and frowning.

Example

You have just completed a patient interview which your supervisor has observed through a one-way mirror. As you join your supervisor, you see him frowning and shaking his head from side to side as he writes on his note pad. He looks up at you, still frowning, and says:

Supervisor: There were a number of problems with that interview. I thought your treatment was quite inappropriate in view of your diagnosis.

UNRESPONSIVENESS refers to inattentive behavior. If someone is unresponsive to you, he does not respond when you talk to him (he may just continue what he was doing). He may avoid eye contact with you, avoid talking to you, and generally ignore you. He simply carries on doing whatever he was doing before you spoke to him. He acts as though you were "not there."

Example

While standing in the hospital cafeteria line, you notice a health professional you met the previous day at rounds. As she walks past you with her food tray, you say, "Hello," but she makes no response and walks on by. You're not sure whether she just didn't hear or see you, or whether she's ignoring you deliberately.

DEPRESSION is expressed by a sad facial expression, tears, sighing, and statements that one feels unhappy.

Example

Mrs. Smith delivered a baby three weeks ago, and this is her first post-partum visit. While you are interviewing Mrs. Smith about her baby, her face looks very sad and she starts to cry.

Mrs. Smith: Oh, I don't know what's wrong with me. Sometimes I feel I just can't cope with the baby. I'm sorry, I don't mean to burden you with my problems (wipes away a few more tears).

IMPULSIVITY refers to sudden inappropriate behavior which may be irrational or immature.

Example

You are examining a 14-year-old when he suddenly says:

Patient: Hey, you wanna hear how good I can belch? (He then belches loudly and smiles proudly.) Pretty good, eh?

AFFECTION is behavior that expresses warmth, caring, or appreciation towards another person. Affection can be expressed by smiling, touching, soft voice tone, and saying things like, "I care about you," or "I like you."

Example

Yesterday you showed Mr. Brown how to walk using

crutches. Today he comes up to you on the ward and, touching your arm, says:

Mr. Brown: Thank you for the help you gave me yesterday. I really appreciated it. (He gives you a warm smile.)

MAKING MISTAKES refers to making an error of some sort. You can make mistakes in front of others or when you are alone. The tension caused by making mistakes often comes not from the fact that other people might disapprove of your mistakes, but from the fact that you disapprove of your poor performance.

Example

While you are leading a tutorial group discussion with other health professionals you mispronounce a word.

You: I'd like to know what the rest of you thing of this patient's myocardial infraction. . . . .uh. . .I mean. . .myocardial infarction. (Thinks: Boy, what a klutz I am.)

No one in the group seems to care that you made a mistake, but you feel foolish nevertheless.

SEXUAL CONTENT refers to words used in conversation to describe sexual behavior or the sex organs.

Example

A male patient says to you: "I think I'm impotent."
You respond by blushing (indicating that sexual content is a stressor for you).

PAIN refers to words, voice tone, facial, or other bodily expressions that patients use to communicate they are experiencing physical pain.

Example

As you are making ward rounds, you pass Mr. Fisher's bed. He says to you:

Mr. Fisher: Please, can you get me something. I feel terrible (moans). My body aches all over. I'm really hurting.

Can you get me something? (Moans again; he is perspiring heavily.)

The first seven stressors—commands, anger, criticism, unresponsiveness, depression, impulsivity, and affection—are derived from the work of Dr. Cliff Christensen. Christensen has identified these seven stressors as being the "troublesome social stimuli" that most often give people trouble. The three additional stressors—pain, making mistakes, and sexual content—have been added because of the research that shows that these three stressors are particularly troublesome for health professionals. Making mistakes may be considered a subcategory of criticism since a person who makes a mistake will often fantasize that others will be critical because of the mistake. These ten troublesome stressors are called INTERPERSONAL STRESSORS because they all involve people acting toward you in a certain way. There are many other forms of stressors that are not interpersonal (e.g., loud street noise caused by traffic).

2. Stressors Can Interfere with Your Work

Health professionals need to know about INTERPERSONAL STRESSORS because some interpersonal stressors are so troublesome that they prevent the health professional from carrying out his job.

Example

Judy is a new member of a community psychiatry team. She has little experience in family therapy and is unsure of the community resources available. During team meetings she would like to speak up but is afraid that she will make a mistake and that someone will criticize her. Result: Judy keeps silent at team meetings, and the other team members begin to feel let down because she isn't contributing. Judy feels anxious during team meetings and depressed afterwards.

In this example Judy's stressor is anticipated criticism. She isn't actually criticized—she only fantasizes making an error and then being criticized. Being criticized is such a powerful stressor for Judy that it blocks her from expressing her opinion and participating in the team discussion. This is summarized in Figure 3.2.

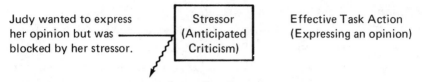

Judy wanted to express
her opinion but was ———— Stressor
blocked by her stressor.   (Anticipated
                             Criticism)

Effective Task Action
(Expressing an opinion)

FIGURE 3.2. Anticipated Criticism is a Stressor

Example

Jim is a health professional interviewing a middle-aged patient, Mr. Wilson, who is attending the clinic because of headaches.

Mr. Wilson: I often get these pains in my forehead.

Jim: When did you last get these pains?

Mr. Wilson: Well, I got them yesterday when I was looking at a picture of my daughter Jane. She died a year ago in a car accident. (Mr. Wilson begins to cry.)

Jim: Crying's not going to help. Try to control yourself!

At this point Jim was feeling very tense and he wanted Mr. Wilson to stop crying. Mr. Wilson's sad face and tears were a powerful stressor for Jim. Jim knew that he should have made a more understanding helping response, but he felt so stressed by Mr. Wilson's sadness that he "lost his cool." Jim became too stressed to function effectively as a health professional with this patient. This is illustrated by Figure 3.3.

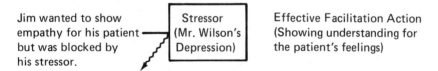

Jim wanted to show
empathy for his patient ———— Stressor
but was blocked by   (Mr. Wilson's
his stressor.   Depression)

Effective Facilitation Action
(Showing understanding for
the patient's feelings)

FIGURE 3.3.   Depression is a Stressor

Example

Yvonne, a health professional student, was seeing a patient who had torn ligaments in her leg while skiing. Yvonne was showing her a muscle strengthening exercise when Jill, Yvonne's supervisor, came by. The following conversation took place:

Jill: Yvonne, you're demonstrating that exercise incorrectly.

Yvonne: What am I doing wrong?

    Jill: See, you exercise the leg this way (moves patient's leg). Don't you pay attention in class?

Yvonne: (Thinks: how can she be so mean. I'd like to tell her what I think of her—but she might get mad at me. That would be awful.)

Yvonne would like to assert herself and confront Jill about Jill's put-down. But Yvonne backs down and keeps quiet because she thinks Jill might get angry at her. Yvonne's fear of anger is so great—that is, anger is such a powerful stressor for her—that it blocks her from acting assertively and standing up for her rights. This is shown in Figure 3.4.

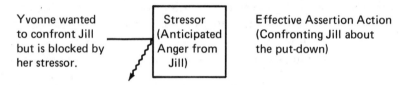

Yvonne wanted to confront Jill but is blocked by her stressor. | Stressor (Anticipated Anger from Jill) | Effective Assertion Action (Confronting Jill about the put-down)

FIGURE 3.4.   Anticipated Anger from Supervisor is a Stressor

These last three examples illustrate how stressors can interfere with a health professional's facilitation, task, and assertion skills—skills that are required to provide effective health care. The point of these examples is that if you want to be an effective health professional, you must be able to cope with interpersonal stress. Knowing what interpersonal skills to use with patients is not enough. You may know how to use a particular skill (such as ACTIVE LISTENING) but be unable to use it with crying patients because you get too stressed. To use the interpersonal skills described in this book you must be relatively free from stress in situations where patients are crying, angry, and so forth. There is no point in your learning any of the action interpersonal skills—facilitation skills, behavior change skills, assertion skills, or problem-solving skills—unless you can also reduce your interpersonal stress sufficiently to be able to use these skills.

Exercise 14:   The Interpersonal Stress Inventory

  Purpose: To identify your interpersonal stressors.

Instructions: 1.   Complete and score the Interpersonal Stress Inventory (shown on pages 89–91) on your own.

2. Look at the scores on your Results Sheet. Circle the highest score you obtained for a stressor in the patient column. Repeat this for the supervisor, student, and $\overline{X}$ columns. The group leader can copy the Results Sheet onto a chalkboard and tally the number of persons who identified a "high score" in each category shown. This will provide a profile of the dominant stressors for the entire group.

INTERPERSONAL STRESS INVENTORY (For Health Professionals)

Instructions: Each item listed below describes a different situation you might experience as a health professional. As you read each item, decide how tense you would feel if you were actually in that situation. Rate how tense you think you would feel using the following 1 to 10 scale.

10	9	8	7	6	5	4	3	2	1
Very Tense		Moderately Tense		Slightly Tense	Slightly Relaxed	Moderately Relaxed			Very Relaxed

Once you have decided on your tension rating, write your rating down in the space provided to the left of the item you are rating.

Your Tension Rating

_____   1. A health professional student frowns at you.
_____   2. A patient is moaning and in pain.
_____   3. A patient criticizes your treatment plan.
_____   4. Your supervisor gives you a command.
_____   5. A health professional student gives you a stern look.
_____   6. You say hello to a patient, but he (she) walks by without noticing you.
_____   7. You make a mistake during a patient interview.
_____   8. A health professional student touches your arm as he (she) says warmly, "Thank you."
_____   9. Your supervisor has a sad look on his (her) face.
_____   10. A health professional student isn't paying attention to what you are saying.
_____   11. A health professional student says, "I like you."
_____   12. A health professional student criticizes your treatment plan.
_____   13. Your supervisor touches your arm as he (she) says warmly, "Thank you."

Your
Tension
Rating

_____	14.	Your supervisor isn't paying attention to what you are saying.
_____	15.	Your supervisor gives you an order.
_____	16.	Your supervisor criticizes your treatment plan.
_____	17.	A patient isn't paying attention to what you are saying.
_____	18.	A patient is holding (his) her stomach and groaning in pain.
_____	19.	A health professional student behaves in an impulsive way while talking to you.
_____	20.	A health professional student shouts at you.
_____	21.	A patient tells you she has a sexual problem.
_____	22.	You receive a low mark on your mid-term test.
_____	23.	You say hello to your supervisor, but he (she) walks by without noticing you.
_____	24.	A patient acts irrationally while talking to you.
_____	25.	A patient gives you a stern look.
_____	26.	A patient says, "I like you."
_____	27.	A patient behaves in an impulsive way while talking to you.
_____	28.	You make a mistake while making your case presentation at rounds.
_____	29.	A patient gives you a command.
_____	30.	A patient touches your arm as he (she) says warmly, "Thank you."
_____	31.	Your supervisor gives you a stern look.
_____	32.	A health professional student gives you a command.
_____	33.	You say hello to a health professional student, but he (she) walks by without noticing you.
_____	34.	A health professional student acts irrationally while talking to you.
_____	35.	A health professional student is crying.
_____	36.	Your supervisor behaves in an impulsive way while talking to you.
_____	37.	A patient tells you he has a sexual problem.
_____	38.	A health professional student has a sad look on his (her) face.
_____	39.	A patient asks you for advice on sexual intercourse.
_____	40.	Your supervisor frowns at you.
_____	41.	Your supervisor acts irrationally while talking to you.
_____	42.	A patient is crying.
_____	43.	A patient shouts at you.
_____	44.	The expression on a patient's face shows he (she) is in a great deal of pain.
_____	45.	A patient has a sad look on his (her) face.
_____	46.	Your supervisor is crying.
_____	47.	A patient gives you an order.

Your
Tension
Rating

——————

————	48.	Your supervisor shouts at you.
————	49.	Your supervisor says, "I like you."
————	50.	A health professional student gives you an order.
————	51.	A patient frowns at you.

RESULTS SHEETS FOR INTERPERSONAL STRESS INVENTORY

Instructions: To score your inventory, add together your tension ratings for the items shown below in parentheses and then *divide the total by 2* (divide by 3 for #8, #9, and #10). This gives you an average score out of 10 for patient, supervisor, and student items corresponding to the same category of stressor (e.g., Anger). For example, if your scores for #29 and #47 were 8 and 6 respectively, then your total would be 14. Divide this total by 2 to get your average score, in this case, 7, which you write in the space provided for the stressor commands.

Add together your *row* totals and divide by 3 to obtain an average ($\overline{X}$) score for each stressor. Next, add together your *column* totals and divide by the number shown in parentheses to obtain average tension scores for patient, supervisor, and student situations (as well as your overall average tension score).

		Tension Rating For			
Stressor	Patient	Supervisor	Student	Total	$\overline{X}$
1. Commands	———— (29+47)	———— (4+15)	———— (32+50)	————	÷3 = ———— 10
2. Anger	———— (25+43)	———— (31+48)	———— (5+20)	————	÷3 = ———— 10
3. Criticism	———— (3+51)	———— (16+40)	———— (1+12)	————	÷3 = ———— 10
4. Unresponsiveness	———— (6+17)	———— (14+23)	———— (10+33)	————	÷3 = ———— 10
5. Depression	———— (42+45)	———— (9+46)	———— (35+38)	————	÷3 = ———— 10
6. Impulsivity	———— (24+27)	———— (36+41)	———— (19+34)	————	÷3 = ———— 10
7. Affection	———— (26+30)	———— (13+49)	———— (8+11)	————	÷3 = ———— 10
8. Making mistakes				———— (7+22+28)	÷3 = ———— 10

Stressor	Tension Rating For				$\overline{X}$
	Patient	Supervisor	Student	Total	
9. Sexual content	_____ (21+37+39)				____ 10
10. Pain	_____ (2+18+44)				____ 10
Total =	____ (÷9)	____ (÷7)	____ (÷7)		____ (÷10)
$\overline{X}$ =	____ 10	____ 10	____ 10		____ 10

Questions for Discussion

- Which stressor did the group score highest on for Patient, Supervisor, and Student items?
- Which stressor did the group score highest on overall? How can this stressor interfere with your being an effective health professional?
- Which role category did the group as a whole experience greater stress with: patients, supervisors, or students?

B. WHAT CAUSES INTERPERSONAL STRESS?

What makes a stressor? That is, why does a social stimulus—like an angry patient—stress one health professional but not another?

Example

Two health professionals, Bill and Jane, are interviewing a patient, Mr. LaPierre, a hemophiliac with a joint bleed.

Bill: Have you been doing the exercises we asked you to do last week?

Mr. LaPierre: Let me tell you about those stupid exercises you gave me! (Mr. LaPierre starts to shout.) I fell down and hurt my arm doing them, and it's all your fault! (Mr. LaPierre glares at them angrily.)

Bill: You're acting rather immature you know! (He glares angrily back at Mr. LaPierre.)

Mr. LaPierre: I didn't come here to be insulted! (Mr. LaPierre gets up to leave.)

> *Jane:* You're really angry because you tried the exercises we recommended and you got hurt. And now you think we're putting you down.
>
> *Mr. LaPierre:* That's right!
>
> *Jane:* Perhaps the exercises were a bit too difficult. Maybe we could find some easier ones for you to do? Could we talk about this a bit more?
>
> *Mr. LaPierre:* Uh . . . well . . . okay. (Mr. LaPierre sits down.)

In this example Bill and Jane respond to Mr. LaPierre's anger differently. Bill becomes so stressed by Mr. LaPierre's anger that he "loses his cool" and acts aggressively towards him. His response is ineffective and only serves to make Mr. LaPierre feel like leaving. Jane, however, remains calm in the face of Mr. LaPierre's anger. She is only slightly stressed by Mr. LaPierre's anger—not enough to interfere with her making an effective response that calms Mr. LaPierre down so that the interview can continue.

Why is the patient's anger a stressor for Bill, but not for Jane? The answer lies in the sort of beliefs or thoughts that Bill and Jane are having as they observe Mr. LaPierre's angry behavior.

Bill's Thoughts	*Jane's Thoughts*
He's angry at *me*.	He's angry at us because he hurt himself.
It's all *my* fault.	It's unpleasant to be yelled at, but I can take it.
This is awful.	How can I help him?
I can't stand it.	
How dare he treat me so badly when I'm trying to help him!	

Bill's thoughts are quite different from Jane's. Bill takes Mr. LaPierre's anger as a personal attack on himself ("He's angry at *me*") and he blames himself. Next, Bill tells himself, "This is awful. I can't stand it." He magnifies the situation—and acts as though it is much worse than it actually is. At this point Bill is feeling very anxious and upset. His bad feelings are a direct consequence of his irrational beliefs ("He doesn't like me. This is awful. I can't stand it."). If you think that something that happens to you is terrible, you're not going to feel relaxed! Like Bill, you'll feel very tense and upset.

The important thing to note here is that Bill's feelings of anxiety, tension, and upset are not caused by Mr. LaPierre's anger.

They are caused by Bill's irrational, catastrophizing beliefs about Mr. LaPierre's anger. What makes Mr. LaPierre's anger a stressor for Bill is not anything Mr. LaPierre does, but what Bill *believes* or *thinks* about what Mr. LaPierre does. If Mr. LaPierre's anger were the sole cause of stress in Bill, then it would also cause stress in Jane. The fact that Jane—although exposed to the same angry patient—doesn't become stressed, shows that it is not the angry behavior that is causing the stress. It is the irrational ideas Bill holds that make him stressed.

Jane has more rational ideas about Mr. LaPierre's anger than does Bill. She doesn't take Mr. LaPierre's anger personally—she realizes that Mr. LaPierre's anger has a specific reason related to the exercises. Jane's belief, that Mr. LaPierre's shouting is unpleasant, is rational and quite different from Bill's irrational belief that Mr. LaPierre's anger is "awful." In addition, Jane rationally concludes that she "can take it"—she realizes that she's not going to be destroyed just because a patient shouts at her. Because Jane's beliefs about the patient's anger are more rational (realistic), Jane is calmer, less stressed. Being less stressed, Jane is able to concentrate her mental energy on thinking of ways to help Mr. LaPierre.

In summary, interpersonal stress is caused by irrational beliefs. This is illustrated in Figure 3.5.

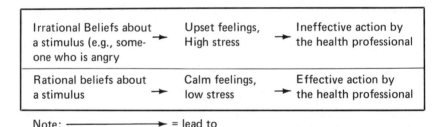

Note: ───────────▶ = lead to

FIGURE 3.5.   Interpersonal Stress Is Caused By Irrational Beliefs

C. HOW TO REDUCE YOUR INTERPERSONAL STRESS

There are three effective techniques you can use to cope with your stressors. They are:

1. POSITIVE COPING STATEMENTS
2. DESENSITIZATION
3. COVERT REHEARSAL

POSITIVE COPING STATEMENTS, DESENSITIZATION, and COVERT REHEARSAL are cognitive reappraisal techniques. They help you to change ("reappraise") your negative, irrational beliefs (your "cognitions") about your stressor. When you eliminate your irrational beliefs and replace them with positive "I can cope" ones, you free yourself to take effective action with patients and other health professionals.

1. Positive Coping Statements

POSITIVE COPING STATEMENTS are positive statements that you can think to yourself when you are becoming stressed. This method of stress-reduction was developed by the psychologist Donald Meichenbaum. Meichenbaum called this approach "stress inoculation" because it prevents stress from reaching a high level. Some general all-purpose coping statements that you can say to yourself are:

> I can handle this.
>
> I can cope with this.
>
> It's not so terrible.
>
> I can stand it.
>
> Everything's going to be all right.

Example

Whenever his supervisor observes him conducting a patient interview, Martin becomes very tense. Martin is so worried that he might make a mistake and get criticized by his supervisor that he ends up conducting a poor interview. During his next patient interview, Martin decides to use positive coping statements to calm himself.

Martin: (Thinks: Oh no, my supervisor is watching me again. what if I blow it? Oh, this is terrible . . . . Just a minute! I'm thinking negative, irrational thoughts again. This is a sign I should start using my positive coping statements. OK, here goes . . . I can handle this. I can cope with this. It's not so terrible if I make a mistake. I can stand it even if I am criticized . . . I can cope with it. I can handle it . . . Everything's going to be all right).

During his interview with the patient, Martin practiced thinking his POSITIVE COPING STATEMENTS several times. As Martin came to focus more and more on his positive beliefs about the situation he felt calmer. The result: Martin conducted a better interview and was later praised by his supervisor.

You can use more individualized POSITIVE COPING STATE-MENTS for specific kinds of stressors. For example, if you find yourself getting angry at a patient or a health professional, you can de-stress yourself by thinking:

Getting angry won't help.

I don't want to lose my temper.

I can cope with this. I can keep calm.

I can stand it—it's not so bad.

Try to understand his point of view.

How can I solve this situation so we both feel good about it?

Notice that along with coping statements specific to controlling your anger ("Getting angry won't help."), you can mix in some of the more general POSITIVE COPING STATEMENTS ("I can cope with this.", "I can stand it.").

The key thing is that you interrupt your irrational beliefs and replace them with your rational POSITIVE COPING STATE-MENTS. "Just a minute," you might be thinking, "what if I don't believe these POSITIVE COPING STATEMENTS I am saying to myself?" If that is the case then you have all the more reason to practice thinking your POSITIVE COPING STATEMENTS. It is because you believe your irrational self statements ("I can't stand it," etc.) that you are stressed. If you concentrate on thinking your POSITIVE COPING STATEMENTS enough times, you will come to believe them. And you will feel less stressed.

To use POSITIVE COPING STATEMENTS follow these steps:

Step 1:   When you find yourself thinking irrational thoughts about a situation, remind yourself to use your POS-ITIVE COPING STATEMENTS.

Step 2:   Think to yourself the general POSITIVE COPING STATEMENTS shown above and any specific coping statements that might apply to your situation.

Step 3:   Repeat step 2 until you feel calmer.

Exercise 15: Designing Your Own Positive Coping Statements

Purpose: To develop skills in identifying your irrational beliefs that make you stressed.

To develop skills in designing POSITIVE COPING STATEMENTS that you can use to reduce your interpersonal stress.

Instructions: 1.   Briefly describe an incident involving another person (patient or health professional) that made you feel very stressed. What did the other person *do* that stressed you? Describe his behavior as accurately as you can.

_____

_____

_____

_____

2.   Classify your stressor by placing a check mark (✓) beside one of the following common stressors:

_____   Commands

_____   Anger

_____   Criticism

_____   Unresponsiveness

_____   Depression

_____   Impulsivity

_____   Affection

_____   Making mistakes

_____   Sexual content

_____   Pain

3.   Identify with a check mark (✓) any of the following irrational beliefs that you might have had in response to your stressor. Be honest with yourself.

_____   If he/she doesn't like me, it's just awful.

_____ If I make a mistake, it's just awful.

_____ This is terrible.

_____ I can't stand it.

_____ How dare he/she act this way.

_____ I'm no good, I'm a louse.

_____ I'm a bad person.

_____ He/she deserves to be punished.

_____ It's hopeless—there's nothing I can do.

_____ Other (please specify): _____

4. Write down five or six POSITIVE COPING STATEMENTS you could think to yourself to reduce your stress in this situation.

(a) _____

(b) _____

(c) _____

(d) _____

(e) _____

(f) _____

Place an asterisk * beside the two coping statements you like best.

5. Discuss this exercise in pairs.

6. The next time you feel stressed by a similar incident, use the POSITIVE COPING STATEMENTS you identified in step 4.

Questions for Discussion

- What irrational beliefs were chosen most frequently by the group?
- What POSITIVE COPING STATEMENTS were selected as the most preferred by the group?

Exercise 16: Practicing Positive Coping Statements

Purpose: To practice your POSITIVE COPING STATEMENTS in response to an actual stressor.

Instructions: 1.   This exercise can be assigned by the group leader as a homework assignment. Each group member, during the coming week, should practice thinking POSITIVE COPING STATE-MENTS in response to an actual stressor. The stressor may either be one experienced (e.g., your supervisor shouts at you) or anticipated (e.g., you imagine your supervisor might shout at you).

2.   At the beginning of the next group session (after one week), divide the class into groups of 4 to 6. Each group member should describe the stressor encountered, the POSITIVE COP-ING STATEMENTS he used, the number of times he used his coping statements, and whether using the POSITIVE COPING STATEMENTS helped reduce his stress.

3.   This exercise can be repeated over several weeks in order to build students' confidence in using POSITIVE COPING STATEMENTS.

Questions for Discussion

- Did using POSITIVE COPING STATEMENTS help reduce your stress?

- How difficult was it to use your POSITIVE COPING STATEMENTS?

- If your coping statements didn't reduce your stress, check to see if you were thinking irrational beliefs instead of countering them consistently with your POSITIVE COPING STATEMENTS.

2. Desensitization

DESENSITIZATION is a technique you can use to build up your tolerance for a stressor. DESENSITIZATION is one of the most widely used and researched techniques for coping with stress. It is a method for making yourself "less sensitive" to an upsetting stressor, such as an angry patient. To DESENSITIZE yourself to a stressor you must expose yourself to your stressor for increasing lengths of time so that you become habituated (used to) your stressor. You learn to "put up with it," so to speak.

Example

Sally, a health professional student, is assigned to a pediatric ward where many children are being treated for leukemia. Part of the treatment for leukemia involves taking a drug that causes hair loss. Sally feels very stressed at first when she sees a five-year-old boy who is completely bald. She avoids looking at him. After she has worked and played with him for three weeks, Sally realizes that she is no longer upset by his baldness.

This is an example of DESENSITIZATION. The strange and frightening becomes familiar and less stressful through repeated exposure. Becoming desensitized doesn't mean becoming less sensitive to the needs of others. By desensitizing yourself to your stressors, you will be freer from stress and able to act more effectively to help others.

To DESENSITIZE yourself to a stressor, follow these steps:

Step 1: Sit or lie in a comfortable position away from distracting noises.

Step 2: For 5 seconds imagine your stressor in detail. You may wish to close your eyes or keep them open while doing this. Imagine that you are in the presence of your stressor. Concentrate on noticing in detail what the person who stresses you is doing. Try to recall as vividly as you can what he says and does that stresses you. As you imagine this, do not try to change the other person's behavior. Your goal is to learn to tolerate this person doing whatever he does that stresses you. After 5 seconds, stop imagining your stressor. If you feel tense that's all right. Your goal is to focus on your stressor and build up your tolerance for it.

Step 3: Think of a peaceful, relaxing scene for several seconds to calm yourself.

Step 4: Repeat step 2 for 10 seconds.

Step 5: Again, think of a peaceful, relaxing scene for several seconds.

Step 6: Repeat steps 2 and 3, each time increasing the length of time you imagine your stressor. Increase your exposure a few seconds at a time until you can imagine your stressor for at least one minute. If you feel very stressed at a particular length of exposure (for example 10 seconds) continue to practice steps 2 and 3 several times at that time interval until your stress reaches a tolerable level. Remember, you don't need to feel perfectly relaxed before increasing your exposure time.

Step 7: Repeat steps 1 to 6 several times a day, and for several days, until you feel comfortable imagining your stressor.

Example

Anna found it very difficult dealing with Mrs. Smith, a new patient on the ward. Whenever she spoke to Mrs. Smith, Mrs. Smith would complain to Anna about not getting enough care. Anna was satisfied that Mrs. Smith was getting good care, but she felt very tense whenever Mrs. Smith complained. Anna felt as though she were being personally criticized by Mrs. Smith. Soon Anna began to dread going near Mrs. Smith's bed. Even the thought of Mrs. Smith's complaining made Anna feel tense. Finally, Anna decided to reduce her stress by DESENSITIZING herself to Mrs. Smith's complaints.

Anna sat in a comfortable chair in her living room (Step 1) and then began the DESENSITIZATION exercise:

Anna: Thinks: Alright, I'm supposed to imagine Mrs. Smith complaining. OK, here goes. I can see myself coming into Mrs. Smith's room, and then Mrs. Smith says, "It's about time. Don't you people work around here? My word, all the money we taxpayers put into health care and we get such dreadful service." Her tone of voice and facial expression are disapproving. She's almost scowling at me . . . OK, that's about 5 seconds (Step 2). Gee, I felt tense but I was able to imagine it! Now to think of something relaxing . . . I'll imagine I'm lying on a tropical beach . . . . There, I can see the palms swaying in the breeze . . . I can feel the warm sand beneath me . . . Calm, very calm (Step 3). OK, now to imagine Mrs. Smith again, only longer. I enter Mrs. Smith's room, and she gives me a disapproving look. (Anna imagines Mrs. Smith complaining.) That's about 10 seconds . . . OK, stop. (Step 2)

Anna continued to imagine her stressor until she could tolerate one minute's exposure. The next day Anna found she didn't feel nearly so tense when she went near Mrs. Smith. Being DESENSITIZED to Mrs. Smith's critical behavior, Anna was now able to remain calm enough to talk with Mrs. Smith about why she complained so much. Mrs. Smith revealed that although she seemed very angry, the cause of this was her underlying sadness because she felt lonely. Anna arranged for Mrs. Smith to be moved to a room shared with a woman her own age. Mrs. Smith quickly made friends with her new neighbor and her complaints stopped. By becoming DESENSITIZED to Mrs. Smith's criticism, Anna was able to become more sensitive to Mrs. Smith's real problem—loneliness. DESENSITIZATION helped free Anna to perform effectively as a health professional.

If you find that you get so tense when you try to focus on your stressor that you just can't get a clear image, you can practice two techniques to distance yourself psychologically from your stressor.

First, imagine the person who stresses you has been filmed and that you are watching the film of his aggressive, critical, etc. behavior being played back onto a large white screen. Move the screen as far back as you want in your imagination—10 feet, 20 feet—as long as you can still see the person's face and hear what he is saying. When you feel comfortable imagining this scene at, say, 20 feet, move the screen to about 10 feet in your imagination. When you are comfortable imagining the scene at 10 feet, you are ready to leave out the screen and imagine you are right there in the person's presence.

A second way you can distance yourself from your stressor is to imagine yourself doing something out of the ordinary while you imagine actually being in the presence of your stressor. For example, you can imagine:

Dancing in a circle around the other person.

Patting a dog on the head.

Pouring tea.

Hitting a tennis ball, etc.

The more novel or humorous the activity you imagine, the more it will dilute the impact of your stressor. Imagining yourself doing something novel, silly, or humorous tends to break up the mental set you normally have that leads to your feeling stressed. Your can imagine yourself doing just about any pleasant activity as long as you don't change your stressor. That is, while you imagine yourself, say, dancing around the person who stresses you, continue to focus on his behavior that stresses you. You can use one, or both, of these "distancing" techniques (adapted from the work of Christensen) to get used to imagining your stressor in small, manageable doses.

Exercise 17:   Practicing Desensitization

Purpose: To desensitize yourself to your interpersonal stressors.

Instructions: This activity can be done two ways. The group leader can desensitize the group as a whole (option 1) or the class can be divided into pairs and group members can take turns guiding their partners through the DESENSITIZATION STEPS (option 2).

Instructions for Option 1 (leader-directed)

1.   Briefly explain the rationale for doing this activity.

2.   Ask each group member to *think* of an incident in which he felt highly stressed by someone who was angry or critical towards him.

3.   Guide the group through the DESENSITIZATION STEPS shown below. Have group members get comfortable in their chairs and close their eyes (or keep them open if they prefer). Instruct the group to imagine the details as you "paint" them. The approximate length of time you should present each scene is shown under the column time (in seconds).

Instructions for Option 2 (pairs)

1.   The group leader should briefly explain the rationale for doing this activity and then divide the group into pairs.

2.   Ask your partner to think of an incident in which he felt highly stressed by someone who was angry or critical towards him.

3.   Guide your partner through the DESENSITIZATION
STEPS shown below.

DESENSITIZATION STEPS

Time	Step	Description
20 (sec.)	1.	"Imagine a peaceful scene, the most peaceful one you can think of (pause). Be in your peaceful scene (pause). You are very relaxed, very calm. Notice how relaxed you feel (pause). Everything is so peaceful. Relax. . . .just relax (pause). You are comfortable, very comfortable. Calm, very calm." (Read this *slowly* and in a soothing voice.)
15 (sec.)	2.	"Now imagine your stressful scene. You're there with the aggressive person. He's really angry and critical. Notice what he's saying to you and how angry or critical he looks. Notice his face, listen to his words. He's putting you down, criticizing you, he seems very angry."
	3.	"Open your eyes. I want you to write down how tense you felt while you imagined this scene. Choose a number from 1 to 10 to rate your tension (1 = very relaxed, 10 = very tense). Write down the number that indicates how tense you felt."
20 (sec.)	4.	Repeat Step 1
20 (sec.)	5.	"Now imagine that your stressful scene has been filmed and it is going to be played back on a large white movie screen. Notice the screen. It is 20 feet away. The projector starts to roll and you can see the light flickering on the screen. The picture of your stressing person appears on the screen. Remember, this is a film—you're not actually there with the person. Notice the picture of this person . . . he's really angry or critical. Notice what he's saying to you and how angry or critical he looks. Notice his face, listen to his words. He's putting you down, criticizing you, he seems very angry."
20 (sec.)	6.	Repeat Step 1
30 (sec.)	7.	Repeat Step 5
20 (sec.)	8.	"This time as you imagine your stressful person, imagine you are dancing around him in a circle while you continue to observe his behavior. Alright, go ahead. You are right there with him and he seems very critical, very angry. You start to dance around him in a circle. Feel yourself dancing. As you dance around him you can still see his face and hear what he is saying. His face looks angry or critical and he is

saying unpleasant things to you. But you are dancing, feel yourself dancing around him."

20 (sec.)	9.	Repeat Step 1
30 (sec.)	10.	Repeat Step 8
20 (sec.)	11.	Repeat Step 1
20 (sec.)	12.	Repeat Step 2
20 (sec.)	13.	Repeat Step 1
30 (sec.)	14.	Repeat Step 2
20 (sec.)	15.	Repeat Step 1
40 (sec.)	16.	Repeat Step 2
	17.	Have group members open their eyes and record their tension rating for Step 17. Have group members subtract this tension rating from the tension rating they made in Step 3. The more a group member's tension rating has decreased from Step 3 to Step 17, the more desensitized the group member is becoming to his stressor.

Questions for Discussion

- How many group members experienced a drop in their tension ratings between Step 3 and Step 17?
- Did having the group leader or your partner "paint" your stressful scene for you, help you to focus more accurately?
- During which step of the DESENSITIZATION exercise did your tension seem to drop the most?

3. Covert Rehearsal

COVERT REHEARSAL is the technique of imagining yourself successfully coping with your stressor.

Example

Andrew, a health professional student, was to give a case presentation on Friday. On Thursday evening, although he had prepared a very thorough case presentation, Andrew found himself feeling very tense as he thought about how things might go on Friday. "What if I blow it and give a lousy presentation," he thought. "That would be terrible." Finally, Andrew decided to reduce his stress by practicing COVERT REHEARSAL.

Andrew: Thinks: I'm going to COVERT REHEARSE giving a successful case presentation. Here goes . . . I'm standing before the class and my instructor . . . I can see myself describing the case in detail . . . everyone is nodding in agreement . . . they like what I'm saying. I finish the case presentation, and I've done a really fine job. Several people come up to me and congratulate me. I did really well!

Andrew found that he felt calmer after COVERT REHEARSAL of his presentation. On Friday he gave his case presentation and felt confident all the way through. Afterwards his supervisor complimented him on the thoroughness of his presentation.

The term covert means "hidden," that is, mental (your thoughts can't be seen). Rehearsal means practice. Hence, COVERT REHEARSAL means mental practice of behavior you want to carry out (but are nervous about doing). As a health professional, you will often know what you want to do to be effective with a particular patient or health professional, but your stressor will block you. If you are anticipating a negative reaction from the other person, you may worry about this so much that you fail to concentrate on what it is you want to say or do. By COVERT REHEARSING what you want to say and do with this other person and imagining a successful outcome, you displace your irrational beliefs about possible negative outcomes. This reduces your stress and helps to build in you the expectation of a positive result. You feel encouraged because you expect success.

To practice COVERT REHEARSAL follow these steps:

Step 1:   Identify what it is that you would like to say and do in the stressful situation you expect to encounter.

Step 2:   Imagine yourself in the stressful situation saying and doing exactly what you want.

Step 3:   Imagine yourself receiving a positive response from the other person(s). Imagine things working out happily for you.

Exercise 18: Practicing Covert Rehearsal

Purpose: To develop skills in practicing COVERT REHEARSAL.

Instructions: 1.   Briefly identify a stressful situation involving a patient or health professional in which you want to take some effective action but are anxious about doing so.

_____

_____

_____

2.   Describe in detail what it is you want to say and to do in this situation. That is, what is the effective action you wish to take?

_____

_____

_____

3.   Carry out your COVERT REHEARSAL. Imagine that you are in the stressful situation. See yourself behaving exactly as you'd like to. Imagine your behavior having a positive result. Repeat your COVERT REHEARSAL 3 or 4 times.

4.   When the opportunity arises, actually carry out the effective action you planned in step 2 above.

Questions for Discussion

- Did you have any difficulty imagining yourself handling your stressful situation successfully? What sort of successful outcome did you imagine?

- How stressed did you feel when you actually carried out your effective action? Were you successful?

The uses of the three stress reduction techniques are summarized in the table below:

Stress Reduction Technique	Use
1. POSITIVE COPING STATEMENTS	To calm yourself prior to encountering a stressor, while you are encountering a stressor, and after you encounter a stressor.

Stress Reduction Technique	*Use*
2. DESENSITIZATION	To reduce your oversensitivity to a stressor. Use prior to, or following, an encounter with a stressor.
3. COVERT REHEARSAL	To develop in you the expectation that you will succeed in coping with your stressor. Use prior to encountering your stressor when you know what it is you want to say and do.

SUMMARY

Extensive research on these three cognitive reappraisal techniques shows that they are highly effective in reducing stress. (If you wish to read more about these techniques and the research evidence for them, you can consult the references for this chapter at the back of this book.) By practicing POSITIVE COPING STATEMENTS, DESENSITIZATION, and COVERT RE-HEARSAL, you will be able to reduce your stress to manageable levels so that you can function effectively as a health professional.

4

Developing Facilitation Skills

A. WHAT ARE
FACILITATION SKILLS?

Facilitation skills are interpersonal skills that the health professional uses to develop a trusting relationship with the patient. A trusting relationship is a relationship between a health professional and a patient in which the patient feels trust for the health professional. He feels cared for, and understood by, the health professional. When a patient thinks you care about him and take the time to understand his feelings and concerns, he will be more likely to trust you, confide in you, and comply with your treatment plan. If your patient thinks that you do not care about him, or that you do not understand his feelings and concerns about the problem that brought him to see you, he may not comply with your treatment plan and may not even return to see you.

Example

John and Mark are two health professionals who work in a family practice clinic. John and Mark are both clinically competent, but they differ in the way they relate to their patients. John never greets his patients by name. He enters the examination room and "gets down to business" right away. John rarely smiles at his patients and avoids talking with them about their feelings about their illness. "My job is to treat patients' illnesses, not coddle them," he says. John's patients frequently complain to the secretary about John's brusque manner. His patients frequently break their appointments and fail to take the medicine he prescribes.

Mark, on the other hand, greets all of his patients by name and gives them a warm smile. When a patient is worried about her illness, he shows her that he understands her feelings and reassures her. "My job is to treat patients' illnesses and the best way to do that is by treating the whole person, including the patient's feelings." Mark's patients often tell the secretary how pleased they are with Mark's quality of care. Mark's patients rarely break their appointments or fail to take the medicine he prescribes.

1. Why Is a Trusting
Relationship Important?

Developing a trusting relationship with your patients is no substitute for good quality of care. If you are warm and understanding towards your patients but are clinically incompetent, your patients are being cheated. The purpose of the trusting relationship is to facilitate the delivery of health care. By developing a trusting relationship with your patients, you enhance the quality of care you give to your patients.

A trusting relationship enhances your quality of care in two main ways. First, it builds trust between you and your patient. When your patients trust you, they are more likely to give you personal information that might aid your diagnosis, be compliant with your treatment, and return to see you for further treatment. Second, by establishing a trusting relationship with your patients, you help to decrease the physiological and psychological stress your patients experience with their illness. When patients are ill, they worry about their illness. They feel weak and helpless. Sometimes they are afraid they might not get better or that they might die. They worry about their ability to take care of their loved ones. If they are hospitalized, they experience a sort of "culture shock" from being suddenly immersed in a strange environment away from their families. They may feel lonely or depressed. These psychological responses to being ill are entirely normal. They are also an important source of stress that drains your patient's energy—energy your patient needs to fight his illness.

If you don't know how to establish a trusting relationship with your patient, he will experience greater psychological stress and will have correspondingly less energy to fight his illness (Figure 4.1).

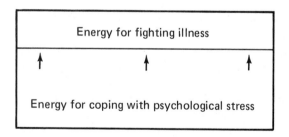

FIGURE 4.1.   Your Patient's Energy When You Fail
to Establish a Trusting Relationship with Him

If you are able to establish a trusting relationship with your patient, he will feel understood and cared for by you. This will reduce his worry and psychological stress so that he will have more energy to fight his illness (Figure 4.2).

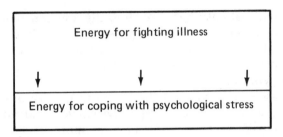

FIGURE 4.2.   Your Patient's Energy When You Establish
a Trusting Relationship with Him

Gerrard (1978) has summarized the findings from 27 experimental studies that investigated the effects of health professionals using a trusting relationship with patients, compared to control groups of health professionals who did not use a trusting relationship. This research shows that when health professionals establish a trusting relationship with their patients, the patients recover quicker, experience less pain, and experience a greater variety of physiological, psychological, and behavioral gains than do patients who do not have a trusting relationship. Korsch (1971), in a detailed study of interviews between health professionals and patients, found that there was no relationship between patient satisfaction and interview length. That is, patients are just as happy with short interviews as they are with long ones. Health professionals do not require "extra time" to practice trusting relationship skills with their patients. You can establish a trusting relationship with your patients in the normal length of time you take for an interview. Most of the trusting relationship skills (such as warmth and active listening) can be demonstrated at the same time as you take a history or perform other "task oriented" functions with patients.

There are two reasons that some health professionals give as excuses for not learning trusting relationship skills: 1) trusting relationship skills may make patients feel better, but they don't actually help patients overcome their illness; 2) busy health professionals don't have the time to practice trusting relationship skills with their patients. Neither of these reasons is supported by the experimental evidence presented above.

2.   Five Facilitation Skills

There are five facilitation skills that you can use to develop ("facilitate") a trusting relationship with your patients. They are:

1. INVITING REQUESTS
2. RESPONDING WITH INFORMATION
3. RESPONDING WITH ACTION
4. WARMTH
5. ACTIVE LISTENING

INVITING REQUESTS is the skill of encouraging your patients to ask you questions or make requests of you. Many patients are afraid to ask questions because they are afraid of appearing stupid or because they think the health professional will get angry. Inviting your patient to request information or action from you is a very facilitative act. Patients really appreciate it.

RESPONDING WITH INFORMATION is the skill of directly answering a patient's question. That is, when a patient requests information from you, you respond by giving the patient the information he wants in language he can understand. Many patients want to know about their illness and its treatment but are reluctant to ask questions. When a patient does ask you a question, it's because it's important to him. You show respect for him by answering his question truthfully. There may be some situations where you will think it inadvisable to give the patient all the information (perhaps because you believe telling him "right now" might be too stressful). In the majority of situations, however, a specific question from your patient deserves a specific, non-evasive answer. If your patient feels you are withholding important information from him, he will not trust you.

RESPONDING WITH ACTION is the skill of carrying out some physical action that your patient has requested. For example, if your patient asks for a drink of water, you could respond by getting it for him. For many people being a patient means being helpless—unable to do for themselves things they normally could do. Patients feel cared for when you help them with their requests for actions they cannot carry out themselves.

WARMTH is the skill of communicating to a patient that you care for him as a person. Being warm means being friendly—smiling at your patient, greeting him by name, showing personal interest in him. WARMTH is a powerful skill for building trust with your patients.

ACTIVE LISTENING is the skill of communicating to a patient that you understand his feelings and concerns. When you AC- TIVE LISTEN to a patient you let him know in your own words that you understand exactly what he is feeling and experiencing. Many helping professionals believe that ACTIVE LISTENING is one of the most important helping skills you can learn.

The five facilitation skills are illustrated in the example below.

Example

A health professional is talking to his patient, a 45-year- old male who was recently hospitalized for a myocardial infarction. The patient is due to leave the hospital to- morrow. The health professional has been telling the pa- tient how to use his nitroglycerine tablets.

Health professional:	If you get chest pain again, take one of the nitroglycerine tablets. Don't swallow it— just hold it under your tongue. There . . . I think that just about covers everything. (Smiles at patient) I'm pleased with how well you've been responding. (WARMTH) You'll be able to go home tomorrow after- noon. Now, are there any questions you'd like to ask me? (INVITES REQUEST)
Patient:	Yes, there are. Uh . . . will it be safe for me to have sex with my wife?
Health professional:	Yes, absolutely. There's no reason why you can't resume your sexual relations with your wife after a few weeks. You should avoid sex, however, during times you are feeling stressed because then it will put an extra load on your heart. (RESPOND WITH INFORMATION)
Patient:	Oh, that sounds OK. (Patient has a puzzled look on his face.)
Health professional:	You have a puzzled look on your face. Per- haps there's something worrying you that we haven't talked about yet. (ACTIVE LISTENS) Is there something else you'd like to ask me? (INVITES REQUEST)
Patient:	Well, this has been worrying me a lot ac- tually. I've never had a heart attack before,

and I'm concerned about the damage to my heart. Does this mean that I'm more likely to die at an earlier age?

Health professional: Not necessarily. Your heart will heal in about 4 months, and you'll be able to resume all the activities you previously enjoyed. If you watch your diet, take your medication, and avoid unnecessary stress at work and at home, you probably won't have any problems. (RESPONDS WITH INFORMATION) I can see that this is something that has been worrying you and that you are afraid that you really won't get better. (ACTIVE LISTENS) That's a normal fear that almost every heart attack patient has. But you needn't worry.

Patient: Thank you.

Health professional: Well, I've got to go now. I'll drop by and see you tomorrow before you leave the hospital. Is there anything else I can do for you? (INVITES REQUEST)

Patient: Could you get me another pillow? When I sit up in bed I keep bumping against the headboard.

Health professional: Sure (goes across the room and brings the patient a pillow). Here you go! (RESPONDS WITH ACTION) (Smiles at patient) See you tomorrow. (WARMTH)

The table below summarizes some basic patient needs, the facilitation responses that health professionals can use to satisfy these patient needs, and the effect of the facilitation responses on patients.

Patient Need	Health Professional's Facilitation Response	Effect on Patient
Information	INVITES REQUEST	The Patient feels
	RESPONDS WITH INFORMATION	cared for, understood, helped. He
Action	RESPONDS WITH ACTION	feels greater trust
To be cared for	WARMTH	in the health professional.
To be understood	ACTIVE LISTENING	

All five facilitation skills—INVITES REQUEST, RESPONDS WITH INFORMATION, RESPONDS WITH ACTION, WARMTH, and ACTIVE LISTENING—are important. The first three facilitation skills—INVITES REQUEST, RESPONDS WITH INFORMATION, and RESPONDS WITH ACTION—are already in the behavioral repertoires of most health professionals. That is, most health professionals already know how to use these three facilitation skills—although they may not be using them as frequently as they could. Because many health professionals lack skills in WARMTH and in ACTIVE LISTENING and because of the experimental evidence that indicates these two facilitation skills may be of great importance in producing positive outcomes for patients (Gerrard, 1978), the rest of this chapter will focus on the development of WARMTH and ACTIVE LISTENING skills.

Exercise 19: Identifying Facilitation Skills

Purpose: To develop skills in identifying different facilitation responses.

Instructions: 1.   This exercise should be done in pairs and discussed with the entire group.

2.   Read each of the patient responses below and classify it according to the type of patient need present. Do this by placing the number indicating the relevant patient need (see list below) in the space provided. For some patient responses, more than one need is present.

```
┌─────────────────────────┐
│     Patient Need        │
│                         │
│  1. Information         │
│  2. Action              │
│  3. To be cared for     │
│  4. To be understood    │
└─────────────────────────┘
```

_____(a) Patient to Health professional: Would you get me a glass of water please?

_____(b) Patient A to Patient B: It really burns me up the way the staff ignore you around here.

_____(c) Patient to Health professional: I feel just terrible. You've got to get me something quick. Please.

_____(d) Patient to Health professional: Why do I have to take these pills?

_____(e) Patient to Health professional: This surgery I'm in here for . . . uh . . . I'm not sure I want to go through with it.

3. Read each of the responses listed below and classify it according to type of facilitation response. Do this by placing the number indicating the relevant facilitation response (see list below) in the space provided. For some responses, more than one type of facilitation response may apply.

```
┌─────────────────────────────────────────────┐
│       Type of Facilitation Response         │
│                                             │
│  1. INVITES REQUEST                         │
│  2. RESPONDS WITH INFORMATION               │
│  3. RESPONDS WITH ACTION                    │
│  4. WARMTH                                  │
│  5. ACTIVE LISTENING                        │
│  6. NOT A FACILITATION RESPONSE             │
└─────────────────────────────────────────────┘
```

_____(a) Health professional to Patient: Hello, my name's Bob Jones. (Shakes patient's hand.)

_____(b) Health professional to Patient: How do you feel about what I've said to you so far?

_____(c) Patient: I've had the flu for a week now. I just can't seem to shake it no matter what I try. I want you to give me some penicillin.
Health professional: It's up to me to decide what medication you get.

_____(d) Patient: Since my husband died there are times I wonder whether it's worth carrying on. The house seems so empty.
Health professional: You really miss him. Sometimes you feel so lonely you feel like giving up.

_____(e) Patient: That term you just used, "otitis media," what does that mean?
Health professional: That's a medical term for what you have—an ear infection.

_____(f) Patient: I'm having trouble walking with these crutches. See . . . . the rubber tip at the bottom has worn away. Can I have a new pair?
Health professional: I see what you mean. They must be quite difficult to use. Here, try these. (Hands new pair of crutches to the patient.)

B. DEVELOPING SKILLS IN WARMTH

WARMTH is the helping skill you use to *show* a patient you care about him. Simply caring about your patient is not enough. You must be able to communicate this caring to your patient if it is to have a tangible effect on him. WARMTH is primarily a non-verbal dimension. It is communicated through your smile, your voice tone, and your physically ATTENDING to your patient. By ATTENDING you demonstrate, through your body posture, that you are paying attention to your patient. ATTENDING is respectful behavior. Through it you show your patient that you care enough about him to focus carefully on what he is saying and doing. ATTENDING is WARMTH demonstrated through your posture.

To ATTEND to a patient you:

1. Sit or stand so that your head is at the same level as the patient's head. That is, you avoid "talking down" to the patient (e.g., you don't stand while the patient is sitting). It may not always be possible for you to get "on the same level" as your patient, but when it is possible, do so. Your patients will appreciate it (especially if they are children).

2. Maintain frequent (but not continuous) eye contact with the patient while you are speaking to him.

3. Face the patient squarely so that your shoulders are parallel to the patient's shoulders. Your face is the most important part of your body for communicating and receiving messages. By "facing" your patient directly you permit optimum communication to occur (Figure 4.3).

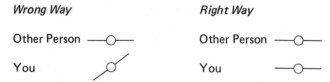

FIGURE 4.3. First Posture Is Not Facing Other Person Directly; Second Is Correct Posture

4. Lean slightly towards the patient. This communicates your interest in what the patient is saying. It's as though you are leaning forward so your ears can catch every word the patient says.

5. Maintain an open posture with your arms. Avoid folding your arms across your chest as this gives the impression you are "closed" to what the patient is saying (Figure 4.4).

FIGURE 4.4. Closed Versus Open Posture

When sitting, place both of your feet on the floor. This is a more open posture than crossing your legs because it is an easier position in which to lean slightly forward.

By ATTENDING to your patient you show him you are interested in what he has to say. By smiling occasionally (for example, when greeting and when leaving your patient) and by speaking in a warm, friendly voice (you avoid sounding uninterested in what the patient is saying), you can add to your ATTENDING skills to show greater WARMTH to your patient. In addition, you can show WARMTH for your patient by what you say to him: greeting him by name, asking how his family is, occasionally showing interest in his interests. You can also communicate WARMTH by touching your patient: shaking his hand when you greet him, giving him a reassuring pat on the arm on leaving.

All of these WARMTH skills make up what is sometimes referred to as "good bedside manner." It is important that you be aware of the many non-verbal ways you can communicate

WARMTH because these non-verbal channels can also be used to communicate "coldness" to your patient.

Example

Elaine, a health professional student, is conducting an interview with a "programmed patient," Mr. Wilson. Mr. Wilson is an actor who is paid to play the role of a patient so that students can get practice interviewing. Elaine's supervisor, together with other health professional students, is watching the interview from behind a one-way mirror.

Elaine:	(Walks into the examination room where Mr. Wilson is sitting. Elaine remains standing.) What seems to be the problem?
Mr. Wilson:	Well . . . uh . . . I've been having this pain in my right arm. It's been bothering me all week, and I thought I better get it looked at.
Elaine:	Could you tell me more about this pain? Where exactly does it hurt, and what sort of pain is it? (As Elaine talks she is writing and doesn't look at Mr. Wilson. While Mr. Wilson describes his symptoms, Elaine continues to write in her notebook and she does not look at Mr. Wilson.)

At the end of the interview, Elaine's supervisor joins Elaine and Mr. Wilson to talk about the interview.

Supervisor:	How do you feel you did, Elaine?
Elaine:	Oh, well, I thought I got most of the history down. I may have missed one or two things, but I think I got most of the information.
Supervisor:	How do you think Mr. Wilson felt during your interview with him?
Elaine:	Uh . . . I don't know. OK, I guess.
Supervisor:	Mr. Wilson, how did you feel about the interview?
Mr. Wilson:	I had the impression she wasn't terribly interested in me.
Elaine:	Oh, dear . . . why did you feel that way?
Mr. Wilson:	Well, when you came in you didn't say hello or anything. Then you spent the whole time writing and

you rarely looked at me. I felt like a piece of furniture!

Supervisor: You thought you were being ignored.

Mr. Wilson: Yes.

Supervisor: How did you feel about Elaine standing while you were sitting?

Mr. Wilson: Well, I felt pretty insignificant. I thought she was about to leave the room most of the time . . . like she didn't have time to sit down and talk to me.

Supervisor: If you were a real patient, would you come back to see Elaine again?

Mr. Wilson: I don't know . . . possibly not.

Elaine: You know, what really surprises me here is that I really did care about you and what you were saying —that's why I made such careful notes. But I hear you saying that you thought I didn't care about you.

Mr. Wilson: That's right.

Supervisor: I can see that you did care, Elaine, but your body language communicated a different message. By standing, writing continuously, and not saying hello, you communicated an impression of coldness and lack of interest.

Elaine: I guess I did.

Exercise 20:   Warm, Cold, Warm

Purpose: To develop skills in recognizing ATTENDING behavior. To experience the effect of having someone attending and non-attending to you.

Instructions: 1.   Divide the group into pairs. For each pair, one member should be "A"; the other "B."

2.   The A's discuss their favorite hobbies for two minutes. During the first 30 seconds, the B's should practice good ATTENDING skills. When A has spoken for 30 seconds, B should show lack of interest in what A is saying by doing one or more of the following:

- leaning backward
- avoiding eye contact

- folding arms across chest
- looking bored
- not facing the speaker

3. After 2 minutes (or sooner, if the A's all stop talking), the group leader should ask each A to describe:

   (a) what his partner did to non-attend.
   (b) how he felt and behaved when his partner ignored him.

4. The A's continue to talk about their hobbies, but this time the B's all practice good ATTEND-ING skills for 2 minutes.

5. After 2 minutes are up, the group leader should ask each A to describe:

   (a) what his partner did to ATTEND.
   (b) how he felt and behaved when his partner AT-TENDED to him.

6. The A's and B's switch roles and repeat the exercise (steps 2 to 5).

Questions for Discussion

- How tense does it make you feel when someone non-attends to you?
- When you non-attended to your partner, were you able to tell if he got upset? Why is it that some health professionals aren't aware of the effect their non-attending behavior has on patients?
- What non-attending behavior by your partner made you most tense?

Exercise 21:   Identifying Attending Behaviors

Purpose: To develop skills in identifying ATTENDING behaviors. To receive feedback on your own WARMTH skills.

Instructions: 1. Divide the group into groups of 4. For each small group, one member should be A, the others B, C, and D.

2. For 7 minutes, A and B should talk to each other about what they like and dislike about being a student (or being a health professional). C and D should move their chairs slightly away from A and B but be close enough so that they can hear and observe what is being discussed. C and D are to act as observers. C should observe A, and D should observe B. Each observer should use the OBSERVATION SHEET (see below) to write down examples of good and poor attending behavior that the person he is observing demonstrates. (For example: "A leans forward, smiles, crosses his legs. His face looks tense, his speech is rapid. Now he is speaking more slowly, his face seems more relaxed"). The observers should focus on the *non-verbal behavior* of the persons they are observing. Comments about what you think the other person is feeling or thinking, or what his motives are, should not be recorded.

OBSERVATION SHEET

Name of Person Observed:_____

Name of Observer: _____
Your observation of the subject's non-verbal behavior (be specific):

_____

_____

_____

_____

_____

_____

_____

_____

3. At the end of 7 minutes, the group leader
    should stop the discussion. C should give
    feedback to A on the non-verbal behaviors C
    observed A making. C should tell A which of
    A's ATTENDING behaviors he liked best. D
    should next give feedback to B on the non-
    verbal behaviors D observed B making. D
    should then tell B which of B's ATTENDING
    behaviors he liked best. Each observer should
    point out when he thought the person he was
    observing ATTENDED well, or poorly.

4. The exercise is repeated, but this time C and D
    discuss the topics while A observes D and B
    observes C.

Questions for Discussion

• Were you surprised by the feedback you received on your
  non-verbal behavior?

• Why are most people not aware of how well they ATTEND,
  or do not ATTEND, to others?

Exercise 22:   Assessing Your Warmth Skills

Purpose: To develop skills in assessing WARMTH. To receive
             feedback on your own WARMTH skills.

Instructions: 1. Divide the class into groups of 4.

2. During the week each group member is to
    make a 10-minute videotape of himself inter-
    viewing a patient. (If patients are not available,
    group members can interview each other about
    a topic of personal significance to the inter-
    viewee.)

3. Each small group meets by itself to view the
    videotapes made in step 2. As the first group
    member shows his videotape to the group, all
    the group members should use the WARMTH
    CONTENT ANALYSIS SHEET (below) to
    check off the WARMTH behaviors they see
    the interviewer demonstrating in the interview.

(WARMTH behavior for the interviewee is not scored.)

WARMTH CONTENT ANALYSIS SHEET

Instructions: Each time you observe the interviewer demonstrate one of the WARMTH behaviors listed below during a *one-minute interval*, place a check mark (✓) in the appropriate column. For example, if during the first minute of the interview the interviewer smiles, has a warm voice tone, and leans slightly forward, place a check mark in the one-minute column beside the rows marked: smiles, warm voice tone, and leans slightly forward. If the interviewer engages in a behavior more than once during a one-minute interval, you still give it only one check mark. That is, during a one-minute interval you are only checking off whether or not a behavior occurs—how often it occurs doesn't matter. When one minute is up (use the second hand on your watch to keep track), move to the next "minute" column and check off in that column any behaviors that occur during that minute interval. During each one-minute interval you will be making a separate set of ratings. When the interview is over (or when 10 minutes is up), add up your check marks in each row and write the total in the last column.

One way to record the interviewer's behavior is to watch the videotape for one minute, then quickly check off the behaviors that you remember occurred. Then watch the videotape for another minute, and again check off the behaviors that you remember occurred, etc. Alternatively, at the end of each one-minute interval, one group member could turn the videotape monitor off for a few seconds while the other group members complete the content analysis sheet for the one-minute interval just viewed.

At the end of the 10-minute interview, after each group member has totaled his scores for his WARMTH CONTENT ANALYSIS SHEET,

each group member should use the WARMTH
RATING SCALE to rate *overall* how warm he
felt the interviewer's behavior was.

Note that these two scales measure different
aspects of WARMTH. The content analysis sheet
provides information on specific behaviors that
occurred during the interview. The rating scale
provides an overall assessment of the quality of
WARMTH provided by the interviewer. (Four sets
of the rating sheets are provided one for each
group member. Remember to rate yourself as
well.) When the ratings are complete, each group
member should give the interviewer feedback
on his WARMTH scores: this feedback includes
the overall WARMTH rating and the specific
behaviors used to communicate warmth. As each
group member completes his feedback, he should
finish by telling the interviewer the one thing the
interviewer did *best* to show WARMTH to the
interviewee.

Repeat the above steps with each group member until everyone has had a turn receiving feedback on his videotape.

WARMTH CONTENT ANALYSIS SHEET

Name of Person Rated:_____ Name of Rater:_____

One-Minute Intervals

Interviewer's Behavior	1	2	3	4	5	6	7	8	9	10	total
1. Maintains eye contact											
2. Faces interviewee "squarely"											
3. Leans forward slightly											
4. Open posture: arms											
5. Open posture: legs											
6. Relaxed posture											
7. Nods head to show interest											
8. Smiles											
9. Jokes											
10. Warm voice tone											
11. Face shows interest, attentiveness											
12. Speech content shows interest											

WARMTH RATING SCALE

Instructions: Place a check mark (✓) in the box beside the rating that indicates how warm you felt the interviewer's behavior was.

4.0	☐	Very good response: very warm
3.5	☐	
3.0	☐	Good response: warm
2.5	☐	
2.0	☐	Poor response: cool
1.5	☐	
1.0	☐	Very poor response: cold

WARMTH CONTENT ANALYSIS SHEET

Name of Person Rated:_____ Name of Rater:_____

One-Minute Intervals

Interviewer's Behavior	1	2	3	4	5	6	7	8	9	10	total
1. Maintains eye contact											
2. Faces interviewee "squarely"											
3. Leans forward slightly											
4. Open posture: arms											
5. Open posture: legs											
6. Relaxed posture											
7. Nods head to show interest											
8. Smiles											
9. Jokes											
10. Warm voice tone											
11. Face shows interest, attentiveness											
12. Speech content shows interest											

WARMTH RATING SCALE

Instructions: Place a check mark (✓) in the box beside the rating that indicates how warm you felt the interviewer's behavior was.

4.0 ☐ Very good response: very warm
3.5
3.0 ☐ Good response: warm
2.5
2.0 ☐ Poor response: cool
1.5
1.0 ☐ Very poor response: cold

WARMTH CONTENT ANALYSIS SHEET

Name of Person Rated:_____ Name of Rater:_____

One-Minute Intervals

Interviewer's Behavior	1	2	3	4	5	6	7	8	9	10	total
1. Maintains eye contact											
2. Faces interviewee "squarely"											
3. Leans forward slightly											
4. Open posture: arms											
5. Open posture: legs											
6. Relaxed posture											
7. Nods head to show interest											
8. Smiles											
9. Jokes											
10. Warm voice tone											
11. Face shows interest, attentiveness											
12. Speech content shows interest											

WARMTH RATING SCALE

Instructions: Place a check mark (✓) in the box beside the rating that indicates how warm you felt the interviewer's behavior was.

4.0	☐	Very good response: very warm
3.5		
3.0	☐	Good response: warm
2.5		
2.0	☐	Poor response: cool
1.5		
1.0	☐	Very poor response: cold

WARMTH CONTENT ANALYSIS SHEET

Name of Person Rated:_____ Name of Rater:_____

One-Minute Intervals

Interviewer's Behavior	1	2	3	4	5	6	7	8	9	10	total
1. Maintains eye contact											
2. Faces interviewee "squarely"											
3. Leans forward slightly											
4. Open posture: arms											
5. Open posture: legs											
6. Relaxed posture											
7. Nods head to show interest											
8. Smiles											
9. Jokes											
10. Warm voice tone											
11. Face shows interest, attentiveness											
12. Speech content shows interest											

WARMTH RATING SCALE

Instructions: Place a check mark (✓) in the box beside the rating that indicates how warm you felt the interviewer's behavior was.

4.0	☐	Very good response: very warm
3.5	☐	
3.0	☐	Good response: warm
2.5	☐	
2.0	☐	Poor response: cool
1.5	☐	
1.0	☐	Very poor response: cold

C. DEVELOPING SKILLS IN ACTIVE LISTENING

Listening skills are the skills you use to listen to what your patient is saying to you. When your listening skills are good, your patient will feel that you understand his concerns and he will feel greater trust for you. If your listening skills are poor, he will think that you don't understand his concerns and you may "turn him off."

There are four types of listening skills.

1. PASSIVE LISTENING

2. ACKNOWLEDGEMENT RESPONSES

3. ENCOURAGERS

4. ACTIVE LISTENING*

PASSIVE LISTENING is the skill of not talking while your patient is talking to you. You remain silent and absorb what he is saying. You avoid interrupting him with what you want to say. You show respect for him by giving him a chance to describe his problem and his feelings about his problem.

ACKNOWLEDGEMENT RESPONSES are vocal sounds like "uh-huh" and head nods that communicate to your patient the message, "Yes, I'm listening to you."

ENCOURAGERS are words, phrases, or sentences that you can use to encourage your patient to tell you more about his problem. Some common ENCOURAGERS are:

"Go on."

"Tell me more."

"What happened then?"

"What did you do?"

"When did the problem start?"

Exercise 23:   Practicing Passive and Responsive Listening

Purpose: To practice, and to observe and experience the effect of, PASSIVE and RESPONSIVE LISTENING.

---

*   This list is derived from Thomas Gordon's *T.E.T. Teacher Effectiveness Training.*

Instructions: 1.   Divide the class into pairs.

2.   Have your partner talk to you for 3 minutes about an incident he once experienced that made him feel really happy. While your partner is talking, you should attend to him without talking at all. Do not give any ACKNOWLEDGEMENT RESPONSES or ENCOURAGERS to your partner. Use PASSIVE LISTENING only. Take special care that you do not nod your head while you are listening. Sit as though you were frozen into one position.

How does your partner react to your PASSIVE LISTENING? Ask him how it makes him feel.

3.   Change roles and repeat step 2 of this exercise.

4.   Have your partner continue to tell you about his incident for an additional 3 minutes. This time listen to him using PASSIVE LISTENING, ACKNOWLEDGEMENT RESPONSES ("uh-huh", head nods), and ENCOURAGERS ("Go on", "What happened next?", "That's incredible."). Do not, however, talk at any length with your partner. Restrict *your* side of the conversation to ACKNOWLEDGEMENT RESPONSES and ENCOURAGERS.

How does your partner react to your RESPONSIVE LISTENING? Ask him how it makes him feel.

5.   Reverse roles and repeat step 4 of this exercise.

How did you react to your partner's use of RESPONSIVE LISTENING skills? Tell your partner how it made you feel.

Questions for Discussion

• What type of stressor did you experience when your partner used PASSIVE LISTENING only with you?

- Which listening skills used by your partner—ACKNOWL-
  EDGEMENT RESPONSES or ENCOURAGERS—had the
  more positive impact on you? Why?

ACTIVE LISTENING is the most important listening skill.
ACTIVE LISTENING is the skill of *understanding* what your patient is saying and feeling, and *communicating* to your patient in
your own words what you think he is saying and feeling. You
reflect back to him his thoughts and feelings.

ACTIVE LISTENING is a two-part skill:

1. First you understand
2. Then you communicate your understanding

Example

Your patient says to you, "Since my amputation, I feel
very weak. My debts are piling up, and I've got a wife
and four kids to look after. I just don't know what I'm
going to do."

First you understand: (You think to yourself: He sounds
worried because he thinks he might not be able to provide for his family.)

Then you communicate your understanding: "I hear you
saying you're worried because you think you might not
be able to provide for your family." (ACTIVE LIS-
TENING)

Your patient: (Thinks: He really knows how I feel!)
"Yes, that's it exactly."

Having understood your patient, you can now move on to
explore solutions to his problem: reassurance that he will get better, suggestions for a special diet and exercise to help him regain
his strength. By taking a few seconds to ACTIVE LISTEN to your
patient, you establish a helping relationship of trust and understanding that facilitates your problem-solving.

When health professionals fail to ACTIVE LISTEN to their
patients' feelings, they usually make one of six common errors.
These "six ways to alienate your patients" are:

1. Playing detective
2. Being evaluative

3. Ignoring the problem

4. Giving premature advice

5. Denying there is a problem

6. Being overly optimistic

Each of these destructive response styles is illustrated in the example below:

Example

Veronica, a 26-year-old patient, came to the health care clinic for treatment of her obesity. (She is more than 100 pounds overweight.) During her interview with a health professional, Veronica made the following statement:

Veronica: "My husband nags me all the time—it drives me crazy!"

Type of Response	What the Health Professional Said	Effect on the Patient
1. Playing Detective	"What do you mean he nags you? When and why does he do this? Explain what you mean by crazy."	(Thinks: Why am I getting the third degree? I didn't do anything wrong.)
2. Being Evaluative	"Well, maybe you're doing something to make him nag you."	(Thinks: Whose side is she on anyway?)
3. Ignoring the Problem	"Let's talk about your diet."	(Thinks: I wish I could talk to someone about my husband. I guess she's just not interested.)
4. Giving Premature Advice	"Nag him back—that'll show him."	(Thinks: Good grief! I already tried that and it doesn't work.)
5. Denying there is a Problem	"Oh, I'm sure he doesn't mean it."	(Thinks: How the hell does she know?)
6. Being Overly Optimistic	"Don't worry—things will work out."	(Thinks: They haven't worked out in five years so why should they suddenly work out now? She's really not interested in my personal problems.)

| 7. ACTIVE LISTENING (Effective Response) | "It sounds like you feel pretty angry about the way your husband is always criticizing you." | (Thinks: Yes, I sure do! She really understands how I feel. Maybe I can tell her some more.) |

The first six responses shown are destructive because they ignore the reality of Veronica's feelings. They give Veronica the impression that the health professional does not accept, or does not care about, her feelings. The effect on Veronica is that she stops talking about her feelings. The health professional has alienated Veronica and missed a chance to explore a significant problem in Veronica's life that may contribute to her obesity.

The ACTIVE LISTENING response is an effective helping response. By ACTIVE LISTENING to Veronica, the health professional demonstrates that she cares enough to really listen to and understand Veronica's feelings. In return, Veronica feels greater trust for the health professional and tells her more about the problems with her husband. When the health professional finally suggested that Veronica's overeating might be related to the stress she feels when she fights with her husband, Veronica agreed. The health professional was now able to use her problem-solving techniques to explore with Veronica ways of reducing conflict with her husband. This example illustrates how you can use ACTIVE LISTENING to get your patient to tell you about personal matters that might have an important effect on your patient's health.

Exercise 24:   Identifying Destructive Response Styles

Purpose: To develop skills in identifying types of response styles that have a destructive effect on patients.

Instructions: This exercise should be done in pairs, and discussed afterwards with the entire group. There are six common destructive response styles that you should avoid using when patients feel upset or want to talk to you about their feelings.

> *Destructive Response Styles*
>
> 1. Playing Detective
> 2. Being evaluative
> 3. Ignoring the problem
> 4. Giving premature advice
> 5. Denying there is a problem
> 6. Being overly optimistic

Below is a statement that a patient might make to a health professional. Following the statement are six destructive responses. For each of the destructive responses given, identify the type of destructive response style it is. Do this by placing the number beside the appropriate destructive response style (see list above) in the space provided.

Situation

Mr. Rodriguez, a 50-year-old businessman, has been admitted to the hospital for coronary by-pass surgery, which is to be performed tomorrow. When you stop by his bed on the ward to talk to him, he says to you:

Mr. Rodriguez: I'm not sure I'm doing the right thing. You know . . . my father had heart surgery six years ago, and he died during the operation.

Responses:

_____(a) "What year was it that he had his surgery?"
_____(b) "Relax, everything is going to be fine."
_____(c) "Well, he may not have died because of the surgery. It could have been something else that happened . . . maybe a mix-up by the anesthetist."
_____(d) "Isn't it about time you made up your mind? Do you want the surgery or not?"
_____(e) "How'd you like to watch some TV? I could wheel a portable in here for you."
_____(f) "Of course you're doing the right thing."

An ACTIVE LISTENING response for this situation would be:

"You're afraid to go ahead with your surgery because you think you might die—like your father did."

An ACTIVE LISTENING response consists of two main parts: a reflection of what the patient is *feeling* and a reflection of the *reason* for the patient's feeling. This "reason" part of an ACTIVE LISTENING response is sometimes referred to as a summary of the *content* of what the patient is saying. Content refers to the facts of the situation about which the patient may also have a feeling.

FEELING REFLECTION + CONTENT REFLECTION = ACTIVE LISTENING

These two components are illustrated in the ACTIVE LIS-TENING response the health professional made to Veronica in a previous example:

Health professional: It sounds like you feel pretty angry (FEEL-ING REFLECTION) about the way your husband is always criticizing you (CON-TENT REFLECTION).

One way to make sure you remember to include both a FEELING REFLECTION and a CONTENT REFLECTION in your response is to use the following formula:

"You feel _____ because _____."

After the words "You feel," state what you think the patient is feeling. Use a feeling word to describe the specific feeling: angry, sad, depressed, anxious, happy, etc. After the word "because," state why you think the patient is feeling the way he does. Another way to put yourself into an ACTIVE LISTENING "frame of mind" is to preface your responses with:

"You're saying _____."

or

"I hear you saying _____."

As you become more proficient at ACTIVE LISTENING, you will want to make your responses in a more natural, unstereotyped way.

Example

Your friend Mark, a health professional student, received a poor grade from his supervisor on his course on the cardiovascular system. Mark says to you, "Damn it, how can he do this to me? All during the course he told me I was doing fine, and now I get a low mark!"

Your formula response: You're saying *you feel* angry *because* he let you think you were doing OK when you actually weren't.

Your natural response: It burns you up when you think he didn't treat you fairly.

As this example shows, you can ACTIVE LISTEN to other health professionals, too. When your colleagues have problems they will appreciate your taking the time to ACTIVE LISTEN to them and understand their feelings. It is just as important to build trust in health professional teams as it is to develop in relationships with patients.

When you ACTIVE LISTEN, concentrate on what the other person is saying and feeling. Ask yourself, "How can I show this person I know what he feels?" Put yourself into the other person's "shoes" and try to see the situation from his point of view. Remember: showing a patient or another health professional that you understand what he feels and thinks doesn't mean you have to agree with what he feels and thinks.

When you ACTIVE LISTEN to a patient, avoid parroting what he has said to you. For example:

Patient: I'm not sure I want to take that needle.

Health professional: You're not sure you want to take the needle. (PARROTING)

Patient: (Sounding annoyed) I just said that!

If you parrot someone, you will irritate him. He will think that you are just repeating what he has said and that you don't really understand him. To show that you really do understand, put your response into your own words.

Patient: I'm not sure I want to take that needle.

Health professional: You're worried the needle might hurt. (ACTIVE LISTENS)

Patient: Yeah . . . it's awfully big!

This is a much better response. The patient feels understood and you are now in a position to explore his feelings further, develop trust, and reassure him.

In most cases, you will only need to ACTIVE LISTEN to your patient once or twice during an interview in order to show him that you understand his problem. In situations where your patient is feeling more distressed, however, you will need to make more ACTIVE LISTENING responses to give him time to trust you and to release his feelings. This doesn't mean that you will need to take a longer interview with your patient. In many situations you will be able to "slip in" your ACTIVE LISTENING responses with whatever activity you are carrying out with your patient.

Example

A health professional is talking with Mr. and Mrs. Venturi about their 12-year-old son Bobby. Mr. and Mrs. Venturi brought Bobby to the health center last week for tests because Bobby had suddenly lost weight and developed dry skin with eczematous patches and had a sore dry red tongue. Urinary sugar and blood sugar tests confirm that Bobby has diabetes.

Health professional:	The results of the tests are in and they indicate Bobby has diabetes.
Mr. Venturi:	What? It can't be! Those tests have to be wrong.
Mrs. Venturi:	Oh no, it's not possible. No one in my family has ever had diabetes.
Health professional:	It's quite a shock for you to learn that Bobby has diabetes and you just can't believe it. (ACTIVE LISTENS)
Mr. Venturi:	The tests—can you do them again?
Health professional:	We already did, just to make sure, and there's no doubt about the results. (GIVES INFORMATION) I can see that it's a real jolt for you and that you're really worried about Bobby. (ACTIVE LISTENS)
Mrs. Venturi:	I don't understand it. I just don't understand it!
Health professional:	You just can't believe it's happening to you. (ACTIVE LISTENS)
Mr. Venturi:	How can we help Bobby? What do we have to do?
Health professional:	We can put him on a special diet, and he will have to take particular care of his skin. Bobby will have to take a special drug called insulin to replace the insulin his

body isn't able to manufacture. That's what's causing his symptoms. (GIVES INFORMATION) You seem quite upset, Mrs. Venturi. (ACTIVE LISTENS)

Mrs. Venturi: I can't bear the thought of my son not growing up normal and having a family like other boys.

Health professional: You're sad because you think Bobby won't be able to get married and have children, and you blame yourself for this. (ACTIVE LISTENS)

Mrs. Venturi: Yes.

Health professional: You needn't worry about that. Bobby can live an entirely normal life—he can have children, participate in sports, really do just about anything any other child can. Did you know many famous athletes have diabetes? (GIVES INFORMATION, RE-ASSURANCE)

Mrs. Venturi: No. (Both Mr. and Mrs. Venturi show interest.)

In the space of two minutes, the health professional has used her ACTIVE LISTENING skills to help Mr. and Mrs. Venturi release their upset feelings and to come to terms with Bobby's diabetes. The health professional's ACTIVE LISTENING to the Venturi's helps them to begin to "work through" and accept their feelings and Bobby's disease. By taking the time to understand the Venturi's strong feelings, the health professional helps them to cope with their distress. Through ACTIVE LISTENING to Mrs. Venturi, the health professional quickly identifies and corrects Mrs. Venturi's erroneous assumption about the effect diabetes will have on Bobby's life. The reason the health professional's reassurance is so effective is because it is based on an accurate understanding of the Venturi's feelings and fears. This accurate understanding is provided by the health professional's ACTIVE LISTENING.

Don't use ACTIVE LISTENING unless you genuinely care about the feelings of your patient. If you don't care, your ACTIVE LISTENING won't sound genuine and the patient will feel put down. However, if you do care about your patient, and care enough to genuinely ACTIVE LISTEN to his feelings, he will feel understood and will feel greater trust for you.

Exercise 25: Active Listening: Identifying Feelings

Purpose: To develop skills in identifying the feelings that underlie a speaker's words. To develop skills in identifying the reason a speaker has a particular feeling.

Instructions: This exercise should be done in pairs, but later discussed with the entire group.

Part I:

For each situation shown below, circle the letter beside the feeling that you think the speaker (patient or health professional) is most likely to be experiencing. You can circle more than one feeling. The first one has been done for you as an example.

Situation 1

A man, age 46, says, "I don't know what to do. My wife is a patient on ward 3. She's had a gallbladder attack, and I just don't know how to help her." He feels:

(a) angry
(b) confused
(c) sad
(d) worried
(e) depressed

Situation 2

A female patient, age 8, hospitalized for an appendectomy, says, "I don't want to stay here. I want to go home. Where's my mommy? Please get my mommy." She feels:

(a) depressed
(b) afraid
(c) annoyed
(d) sad
(e) angry

Situation 3

A male patient, age 62, says, "My wife died last week. She died peacefully though. Thank God for small mercies." He feels:

(a) resigned
(b) irritated
(c) relieved
(d) sad
(e) afraid

Situation 4

A female patient, age 25, says, "I didn't have any pain last night. It was the first good night's sleep I had in a week!" She feels:

(a) confused
(b) joyous
(c) happy
(d) agitated
(e) relieved

Situation 5

A male patient, age 9, says, "Do I have to take that needle? It's so big." He feels:

(a) confused
(b) angry
(c) sad
(d) irritated
(e) nervous

Situation 6

A health professional says, "What's the matter with her anyway? I rescheduled this patient's appointment and gave up part of my lunch hour to meet her. You'd think she'd have the courtesy to phone if she's not coming!" He feels:

(a) confused
(b) angry

(c) nervous

(d) sad

(e) afraid

Situation 7

A hospitalized patient, age 35, says, "I really don't like to complain, but I wish you wouldn't ask me if I want my bedpan when I have visitors." She feels:

(a) angry

(b) sad

(c) embarrassed

(d) afraid

(e) nervous

Situation 8

Father of a male patient, age 5, says, "What do you mean my son has diabetes? That can't be right. Please check your tests—there must be a mistake." He feels:

(a) angry

(b) sad

(c) nervous

(d) confused

(e) shocked

Part II:

For each situation shown below, write down as many feeling words as you can think of that describe how you think the speaker is feeling. The first one has been done for you as an example. For the time being, ignore the word "Because" under each feeling response space.

Situation 9

A female patient, age 28, says, "I took the sulfa drug you prescribed for me last night at 10 p.m. After about two hours, I got a real headache and my face started to swell. I've been vomiting all night and I still feel pretty nauseous. Now my hands and feet feel numb. I don't know what's happening so I thought I should come over and see you right away."

She feels: worried, scared, afraid, nervous, anxious

Because: her medication is having strange side effects

Situation 10

A hospitalized patient, age 30, says, "Hey, are there any quiet rooms in this hospital? That patient in the bed next to mine was in and out of bed all night. He was so noisy I hardly got any sleep!"

He feels: _____

Because: _____

Situation 11

A female patient, age 47, says, "Do I really need this x-ray? I've heard that too many x-rays can be very dangerous, and I had a chest x-ray only 6 months ago."

She feels: _____

Because: _____

Situation 12

A hospitalized male patient, age 16, says, "I can go home tomorrow? Fantastic! I never thought I'd look forward to going back to school!"

He feels: _____

Because: _____

Situation 13

A female health professional says, "I was there when she had her baby. It was stillborn. I wanted to do something to help, but there was nothing I could do."

She feels: _____

Because: _____

Situation 14

Mother of male patient, age 8 months, says, "This diaper rash doesn't seem to be clearing up. I don't know what I could be doing wrong. I apply all sorts of creams, but nothing seems to work. I don't know if it's the way I'm washing his diapers or what!"

She feels: _____

Because: _____

Part III:

In part 2 of this exercise you wrote down the feelings you thought the speaker was experiencing. Go back over situations 10 to 14 and write down, following the word "Because," *why* you think each speaker feels the way he or she does. The first one has been done for you as an example.

Exercise 26:   Writing Active Listening Responses

Purpose: To develop skills in writing ACTIVE LISTENING responses.

Instructions: Group members should write their responses by themselves. At the end of the exercise, the group leader can debrief the exercise by having different group members write their responses on a chalkboard to facilitate group discussion.

Part I:

For each of the situations shown below, write an ACTIVE LISTENING response using the "You feel _____ because _____" format. Imagine that the person you are responding to is your patient (or a health professional you know). The first one has been done for you as an example. For the time being, ignore the section marked "Natural Style."

Situation 1

A female patient, age 27, says, "My first child was retarded. I'd like to have another child. But . . . . what if he or she turns out to be retarded as well?"

Your response: You feel worried because you're afraid your next

child might be retarded.

Natural style: You want another child but you're afraid he
might be born retarded. That scares you.

Situation 2

A male patient, age 44, says, "You want to know if I have any stress at home? Oh boy! I got this 16-year-old daughter who doesn't show me any respect. She's on the phone all the time. She's always yelling at her mother. And the way she dresses—you should see the way she dresses. It's a wonder my wife didn't have a heart attack as well."

Your response: _____

_____

Natural style: _____

_____

Situation 3

A female patient, age 75, says, "Oh, I feel much better. The medication really helped. You don't know how wonderful it is not to have that pain anymore."

Your response: _____

_____

Natural style: _____

_____

Situation 4

A male patient, age 7, whose arm you are trying to remove stitches from, says, "Ouch, that hurts!" (Pulls arm away and glares at you.)

Your response: _____

_____

Natural style: _____

_____

Situation 5

Jane, a female patient, age 23, recently had a radical mastectomy of her left breast after a biopsy revealed the presence of a malignant tumor. As you are asking her how she is feeling, she starts to cry.

Your response: _____

_____

Natural style: _____

_____

(Situations 6 and 7 are a continuation of Situation 5).

Situation 6

Jane says, "Why did this have to happen to me? What did I do to deserve this?"

Your response: _____

_____

Natural style: _____

_____

Situation 7

Jane says, "I don't know how my boyfriend's going to react to me."

Your response: _____

_____

Natural style: _____

_____

Situation 8

A health professional you have been working with says: "I just discovered I gave one of my patients a drug she's allergic to. I made an error in checking out her allergy history and prescribed a sulfa drug. She got really sick and had to come in to see me this morning. She was very polite to me, but I really didn't deserve it. I really blew it!"

Your response: _____

_____

Natural style: _____

_____

Part II:

Now rewrite your ACTIVE LISTENING responses, this time using a more natural style. The first one has been done for you as an example.

Exercise 27:   Practicing Active Listening in Pairs

Purpose: To develop skills in practicing ACTIVE LIS-TENING.

Instructions: This exercise should be done in pairs. Each pair will need a token (a poker chip, a pen, a penny, or some other object that can be easily held).

Part I:

Step 1:   Sit facing your partner. Choose a health care topic that you both *disagree* on: for example, abortion, mercy-killing, etc. One of you should take the "For" position; the other should take the "Against" position.

Step 2:   Each of you should take turns defending and explaining your position, but follow this important rule:

Only the person holding the token can express his opinion on the topic. You cannot have a turn explaining your position until you accurately summarize to your partner what your partner has just said and "earn" the token from him.

Let your partner start explaining his position on the chosen topic first. He should hold the token in his hand. After he has spoken for a few minutes, ACTIVE LISTEN to what he has said. Summarize both the content of his words and what you think your partner feels. If your partner agrees that you made an accurate ACTIVE LIS-TENING response to him, he should give you the token as a sign that you did a good job ACTIVE LISTENING to him. It is now your turn to express your opinion. You explain your position while your partner ACTIVE LISTENS to you. When your partner makes an accurate ACTIVE LISTENING response to you, give him the token and switch roles again. Remember, you don't get your turn at talking about your position on the topic *until* you ACTIVE LISTEN *to the other person's satisfaction* and receive the token. The person being ACTIVE LISTENED to is the final judge of whether he was given an accurate ACTIVE LISTENING response. Remember: you are not allowed to express your opinion until you have earned the token from your partner by ACTIVE LISTENING to him.

Example

Jim: I can't stand mercy killing. I think it's a crime against humanity. I just don't understand how any health professional could be for mercy killing.

Judy: I hear you saying you really disapprove of mercy killing. It just doesn't make any sense to you why anyone would advocate mercy killing (ACTIVE LISTENS)

Jim: That's right.

Judy: Did I summarize what you said and felt accurately?

Jim: It was pretty close. (Gives Judy the token.)

Judy: OK, it's my turn now. I support mercy killing because I don't think people should have to suffer continual pain when there's no hope for them. For them, mercy killing is something that they want. It's an act of kindness.

Jim: OK, I hear you saying that you think mercy killing is good because it puts people out of pain. (Attempts ACTIVE LISTENING.)

Judy: No, that's not quite it. What I'm saying is that when there is no hope for someone, when all the doctors agree that someone's life cannot be saved, and that person is in great pain, then mercy killing is a good and desirable thing.

Jim: You're saying you support mercy killing in situations where there's no chance a person will live and his final days are ones of extreme pain. (ACTIVE LISTENS)

Judy: You got it that time! It's your turn now. (Gives Jim the token.)

Step 3:   After 10 minutes, stop and talk about how you feel about doing the exercise. Do you and your partner feel you've understood each other? If your partner is feeling angry or defensive, it's probably because you didn't ACTIVE LISTEN well enough to make him feel understood. If you are both calm and the discussion hasn't "overheated," then you've both probably done an excellent job of ACTIVE LISTENING to each other.

What happens when most topics like the ones you've been discussing are discussed and people don't take time to understand each other?

If you ever have a fight or disagreement with a friend or another health professional and you can talk him into trying the above exercise with you—using your disagreement as the topic—you can improve things between you pretty fast. Try it and see!

Part II:

For this ACTIVE LISTENING exercise you will need 10 poker chips or 10 pennies.

Step 1:   Sit facing your partner. Your partner talks for 15 minutes about an incident that he has strong feelings about and which occurred either recently or in the past. Your partner should hold the poker chips (or pennies) in one hand while he talks to you.

Step 2:   While your partner is telling you his story, ACTIVE LISTEN to him as frequently as you can. Each time that your partner feels you have made an accurate ACTIVE LISTENING response to him, he should give you one poker chip (or penny). The poker chip is feedback to you that you made a good response. See if you can "earn" all 10 poker chips before the 15 minutes are up.

Step 3:   Reverse roles. This time you talk and dispense poker chips while your partner ACTIVE LISTENS to you.

Step 4:   At the end of the exercise, share your feelings about what it's like to be given a poker chip each time you make a good ACTIVE LISTENING response. Does it help you to make better ACTIVE LISTENING responses?

Exercise 28:   Group Exercise in Active Listening

Purpose: To develop your skills in practicing ACTIVE LISTENING. To receive feedback on your ACTIVE LISTENING.

Instructions: This exercise is adapted from an exercise used by Dr. R. Carkhuff. This exercise is best done with a group of 5 to 10 persons.

Part I: Summarizing Content

Step 1:   One person acts as a helpee who has a problem. This person is called the helpee because he would like some help and understanding for his problem. A second person acts as a helper. He is to listen to the helpee and then make a *single* ACTIVE LISTENING response to the helpee. The helper and the helpee should be chosen by having group members volunteer for the roles. Both the helper and the helpee should sit facing each other, slightly away from the rest of the group—but close enough so everyone can hear their conversation.

Step 2:   For 3 minutes, the helpee should talk about a problem he once experienced. It may be a recent problem or one that occurred in the past. It should be an incident in which he experienced strong feelings of some sort, (for example: anger, hurt, sadness, worry, upset, etc.) While the helpee speaks, the helper listens and attends without talking.

Step 3:   At the end of 3 minutes, the helpee should stop talking. If necessary, the group leader can ask the helpee to stop when 3 minutes are up. The helper should wait 1 minute before replying and then summarize to the helpee what the helper thinks the helpee was saying. The helper can do this by saying, "I hear you saying . . . ." or "You're saying that . . . ." and then making his summary. The helper should concentrate on summarizing the content of what the helpee has said and not worry about summarizing what he thinks the helpee *felt* at this time.

During Step 2 and the 1-minute interval of Step 3, the rest of the group should write down their own "I hear

you saying . . . ." summaries of what they thought the
helpee was saying. This is done to give everyone practice
in writing a response. Note that only the other group
members write down their responses; the helper must
formulate his response in his head.

Step 4:   After the helper summarizes what the helpee has said,
each group member should evaluate how accurate the
helper's summary was. If someone thinks the helper's
summary was, on the whole, accurate, he should write
down "Yes" on a piece of paper. If he thinks the helper's
summary was, on the whole, inaccurate (especially if
something really important was left out), he should write
down "No." Writing your evaluation down is important
because people often change their evaluations when they
hear other people's evaluations.

Step 5:   The group leader should ask the helper to evaluate how
accurate he felt his summary was.

Step 6:   The group leader asks the group members who wrote
"Yes" (that the helper's summary was accurate) to raise
their hands. Next, the group leader asks the group members who wrote "No" (that the helper's summary was not
accurate) to raise their hands. The group leader should
share his own evaluation along with the other group
members. Group members who wrote "No" should explain why they felt the helper was inaccurate. This feedback is very helpful in directing helpers to things they
overlooked in their summaries.

Step 7:   The group leader asks the helpee to evaluate how accurate the helper's summary was.

Step 8:   Finally, the group leader asks 3 other group members to
read out the summary statements they themselves wrote
down. After all 3 responses have been read, the group
leader should ask the helpee to choose which summary of
the 3 he liked best, and why. If the helpee says that all of
the responses were good (because he doesn't want to play
favorites) he should be encouraged to choose the one that
was slightly better. This will help the group to identify
what an excellent summary sounds like.

The steps in this exercise may be summarized as follows:

(3 Minutes)   1. Helpee talks, Helper listens. Group writes summaries.
(1 Minute)   2. Helper formulates summary. Group writes summaries.
               3. Helper makes summary.
Feedback: 4. Group rates helper.
               5. Helper evaluates self.
               6. Group evaluates helper.
               7. Helpee evaluates helper.
               8. Three group members share summaries.
               9. Helpee chooses best summary.

Part II: Summarizing Content and Feeling

After each group member has had a chance to make a single content summary as a helper, *this exercise can be repeated* (Steps 1 to 8) with helpers making single ACTIVE LISTENING responses. That is, this time the helper listens to the helpee and then makes a single response summarizing both the *content* of what the helpee has said and the helpee's *feeling.* The helper should respond using the format, "You feel _____ because _____," or "You felt _____ because _____ ."

Part III: Extended Active Listening

After each group member has mastered making a single ACTIVE LISTENING response in Part II, the group will be ready to try making extended ACTIVE LISTENING responses. The same exercise (Steps 1 to 8) is repeated, but with these changes:

1. The helper talks about his problem (or incident that he had strong feelings about) for *15 minutes.*

2. The helper does not wait until the 15 minutes are up to make his ACTIVE LISTENING responses, but ACTIVE LISTENS as many times as he wishes during the helpee's story. Helpers should try to make at least three ACTIVE LISTENING responses during the 15 minutes.

3. The rest of the group should rate how well they feel the helper did, overall, using the ACTIVE LISTENING RATING SCALE (shown on page 176).

Ratings should be written down, just as the "Yes", "No" evaluations were written down previously. Ratings can be given for the mid-points of the scale. For example: 1.0   1.5   2.0   2.5   3.0   3.5   4.0.

Rating	ACTIVE LISTENING RATING SCALE
4	Response accurately reflects deeper feelings and concerns experienced by the speaker. Responses show an understanding of underlying feelings not directly expressed by the speaker.
3	Response accurately reflects the surface feeling of the speaker and summarizes essential content (Minimum ACTIVE LISTENING Level).
2	Response accurately summarizes content but misses the speaker's feelings.
1	A hurtful or destructive response. Ignores or detracts from what the other person has said or is feeling.

When the group members give their evaluations, the leader should write their ratings down on a chalkboard so that everyone can see how the helper was rated. When the helper evaluates himself, and the helpee evaluates the helper, their evaluations should be made using ratings. That is, the helper should state what level he thinks he achieved on the ACTIVE LISTENING rating scale. In addition to rating the helper, the helpee should state what he liked and what he didn't like about the helper's responses.

4. During the exercise, the rest of the group should write down their own ACTIVE LISTENING responses to what the helpee is saying. At the end of the exercise, the group leader should ask three group members to share their best responses. That is, each of the three members selected should read out the one ACTIVE LISTENING RESPONSE he wrote that he felt was his best. The helpee should choose the best of the three and explain why.

The steps in this extended ACTIVE LISTENING exercise are:

(15 minutes)   1. Helpee talks, helper ACTIVE LISTENS. Group writes ACTIVE LISTENING responses and rates helper.

Feedback: 2. Group rates helper's performance *overall* using rating scale.

3. Helper evaluates self.

4. Group evaluates helper.

5. Helpee evaluates helper.
6. Three group members share their best ACTIVE LISTENING responses.
7. Helpee chooses best response.

Questions for Discussion

- When someone ACTIVE LISTENS to you, what effect does it have on you?
- What difficulties did you experience in trying to ACTIVE LISTEN to your helpee?

SUMMARY

Facilitation skills are the interpersonal skills used by the health professional to develop a relationship of trust with patients. Five important facilitation skills are: INVITING REQUESTS, RESPONDING WITH INFORMATION, RESPONDING WITH ACTION, WARMTH, and ACTIVE LISTENING. There is experimental evidence that when health professionals use facilitation skills their patients experience a number of positive physiological, psychological, and behavioral outcomes. By using facilitation skills, health professionals can enhance the quality of care they deliver to patients.

5
Developing Skills in Behavior Change

A. HEALTH
PROFESSIONALS
AND CHANGE

Health professionals are continually faced with change. It occurs on many different levels. As scientific knowledge expands, health professionals must not only keep abreast of these advances, but also find new ways to apply the knowledge to health issues. Governmental, institutional, and agency policies relevant to health care practice change. Roles of existing health professionals are in flux, and innovative educational programs are preparing new types of health care workers. These changes mean that established and new kinds of health professionals must find new ways to work together to meet patient needs.

On the one hand, health professionals themselves need to adapt to changes that affect concepts, policies, and ways of relating to other health care workers. On the other hand, however, part of the role of a health professional is to motivate patients to change unhealthy patterns of living. Thus the health professional who understands change theory and behavioral change principles is better equipped to manage the change he will be involved in.

Example

A variety of health professionals from different departments worked every afternoon in the outpatient specialty clinic. Many of the staff members smoked freely in the corridors, the lab, and in the conference area. The team leader decided that this was unacceptable behavior for several reasons and set about instituting a new policy that would limit smoking to the lounge. The new policy was posted on the bulletin boards, and a copy was sent to each staff member. Over a week's time, she spoke to the individual team members, requesting their cooperation. There was much reluctance, but most agreed to cooperate. The clinic director, a smoker, responded with "Good Luck" but would not commit himself. The first week, there was good cooperation. Only a few staff members smoked in the corridor. The clinic director continued to smoke freely. By the third week, there was smoking in all areas again.

Response A

By the end of the third week, the team leader was angry with the smokers and also with the non-smokers for not exerting peer pressure on the smokers to stop smoking. She was discouraged because the new policy had not changed anyone's behavior and felt personally defeated. She was afraid to bring up the topic again and worried about her adequacy as a team leader.

Response B

The team leader expected resistance to the new policy and accepted staff reluctance as a normal response to change. She focused on their interest in cooperating. She recognized the clinic director as a key motivating force for the rest of the staff and planned to approach him at specific intervals to enlist his cooperation. She accepted the fact that it would take time for the smoking behavior to change. When smoking began again, she did not see it as a personal failure but rather as a signal to institute another approach.

Discussion

In Response A, the team leader reacted personally and felt defeated because her new policy did not change behavior. Her sense of failure in this situation would clearly have an effect on her willingness to institute change in the future. In Response B, an understanding of change theory made it possible for the team leader to anticipate the different stages the staff would pass through before the changed behavior became the pattern. She gave encouragement to staff for smoking in the lounge to reinforce the new behavior. She planned to enlist the cooperation of the clinic director, who was a key staff member. She accepted the fact that change is always difficult and did not take any failure to cooperate as a personal defeat. She was able to deal with the situation objectively and realistically.

B. WHAT IS CHANGE?

Change is a process by which alteration occurs in a system's general structure or function. The introduction of antibiotics, for example, dramatically altered disease management on many different levels. Suddenly, diseases that had frequently been lethal were handled by community physicians on an outpatient basis, and successfully so. Hospital administrators were faced with empty beds, and there had to be a redistribution of resources. It is easy to see that a single change can often precipitate many others.

C. WHAT IS BEHAVIOR CHANGE?

Behavior change refers to an alteration in an individual's or group's reaction(s) to his or its environment. Since none of us exists in a vacuum, we are constantly interacting with other individuals or groups. A change in our behavior will cause change in others if we have contact with them. Different people respond differently to change. Some may like the change and decide to implement the same behavior change in themselves. Others could be very resistant, dig in their heels, and throw all their energy into attempting to counteract the change.

Example

A new department chairman has recently been appointed. Since he comes from another region, he is relatively unknown by department members other than those who served on the selection committee.

Shortly after his arrival, he calls a department meeting. He is very aware of group dynamics and watches to see how the other members react. He first watches seating arrangements and postures assumed by the staff. It quickly becomes obvious where sub-groups are, and as the meeting begins, it becomes obvious that certain groups have met prior to this large group. The purpose of their prior meetings was to consolidate strength in order to defend their particular program if it became necessary. It is also apparent that some department members are anxious for a change in the way the department is run. It is the job of the new department chairman to motivate this group and initiate change in a direction that is acceptable to most of those present.

In order to facilitate change and provoke behavior change, it is essential that the department chairman be familiar with change theory.

D. CHANGE THEORY

In order for a system to change, there must be an introduction of something new. This may be a pattern of behavior, a new attitude or value, or a new concept or idea. When you set out to actively produce change in a group, it is important to realize that the group is maintaining its present way of functioning for a reason. It is committed to that method of operating and may see no reason to alter its function. In other words, the group members will resist learning something new (RESISTANCE).

If you plan to change their operation by teaching them another way of functioning, you must first motivate them to change their present "modus operandi." This requires an unlearning of their usual way of functioning.

PLANNED CHANGE = UNLEARNING PRESENT WAYS OF DOING THINGS

Beware!! The unlearning is not easy, but it can be done. For change to occur the individual or group must proceed through an orderly progression of stages. The model of planned change might be based on the following stages:*

1. motivation
2. changing
3. assimilation

Stage 1: Motivation

Change can only occur if the individual within the system feels it's safe to give up his old responses and learn some new ones. Unless this feeling of psychological safety is present, he will become increasingly defensive.

Example

A public health agency has undergone many staff changes recently and several new graduates have been hired. These people show great potential but at the moment they need much support from older, more mature staff. There have also been policy changes recently which have aggravated those persons with seniority. The general climate in the office is stormy.

As if that's not enough, the director of health announces that the public health staff must teach a health and fitness course in the schools. This is to start in September. It is now July.

The more that changes occur, the less safe the environment will seem and the more the staff will strive to feel secure.

* This has been adapted from work by Lewin and Schein.

The first stage of change is creating the motivation to change. This occurs when threats are withdrawn sufficiently to make the climate psychologically safe. It also requires that the individual's present beliefs, values, and behavior patterns be neither accepted nor rejected. Finally, the actual must be compared with the ideal to provoke a desire for change in the individual.

Using the previous example: The younger staff must feel confident in their skills, and the senior staff must feel respected. The total group must be aware of doing an average job—not poor, not superb. If it were superb, why change? If it were poor, there'd be no sense of safety. The staff must be aware that their status in the community and schools will give more strength to the program and a sense of importance to themselves.

Stage 2: Changing

Group members begin to develop new beliefs, values, and behavior patterns based on new information that is obtained. They actively try to behave in ways that will be rewarded or confirmed. This searching behavior can follow one of two patterns, or a combination of both. First, group members may seek a model on which to model their behavior or program. For example, using the public health situation, the staff could utilize a program which had been successful in an adjoining county. Secondly, they could develop an original program, based on the individual skills of the group members. Or they could develop a personalized program that met the individual needs of the children in their county. Thirdly, they could combine the two models.

The first approach, MODELING, is a simpler, faster alternative but there may be important differences between the group for whom the program was developed and the group about to receive it. Thus, the model may not work.

The latter approach requires more time but it is more likely to be integrated because it meets the unique needs of the community. It is important when changing to select an approach that meets the particular needs of the system.

Stage 3: Assimilation

Assimilation occurs when the new beliefs, attitudes, and behavior patterns are stabilized and integrated into the personality of the individual attempting the change. If the group member is to retain this response, he must receive positive feedback from persons important to him.

Using the public health example, if the staff organize, or adapt, a program and get very positive feedback, they are likely to repeat the program. If the individuals feel good about how they handled the situation, this will reflect on their self-concept and enhance it. If the total group feels good about the outcome, then this is enhancing to the agency. And if the community is pleased and positive outcomes (e.g., better personal hygiene in school students) are apparent, then the change will be assimilated and repeated.

E. WHAT ARE CHANGE STRATEGIES?

There are various strategies that can be used when planning change. Bennis et al. (1976) list three types of strategies for changing: (1) the EMPIRICAL-RATIONAL, (2) the NORMATIVE-RE-EDUCATIVE, and (3) the POWER-COERCIVE. There are fundamental assumptions underlying each of these strategies.

1. Empirical–Rational Strategy

The EMPIRICAL-RATIONAL strategy assumes that people are rational and motivated by self-interest. Therefore, if the proposed change can be rationally justified, and if it can be shown that those involved will gain by the change, the proposed change will be adopted.

Example

A health professional has completed a careful history on a 43-year-old woman. Her diet includes many foods that contain sugar, such as cakes, candy, and soda. She leads a sedentary life. Her physical examination shows her to be overweight.

Health professional: You are in good health except for the fact that you are about 15 pounds overweight and you're not getting enough exercise. These two factors make you more prone to certain medical problems. You would improve your health and feel better if you ate a more careful diet and exercised more.

The health professional went on to give more specific details.

Discussion

The health professional made two basic assumptions: (1) that the patient is rational and (2) that the patient will be motivated to change behavior once the benefit of change is revealed to her. The health professional identified the problems (overweight, too little exercise), provided rationale for change (prevent medical problems, improve health, feel better), and proposed changes (diet, exercise) that were desirable, effective, and in the best interest of the patient. Because rationale had been provided and benefit to the patient described, the health professional assumed that the proposed changes would occur. This illustrates the EMPIRICAL-RATIONAL strategy.

2. Normative–Re-Educative Strategy

The NORMATIVE–RE-EDUCATIVE approach to change sees people as active and in pursuit of impulse and need satisfaction. This approach assumes that their actions are influenced by social and cultural norms and their commitment to these norms. An individual's actions are influenced by his attitude and value systems, which support the socio-cultural norms. Changes in this approach involve change in values, attitudes, skills, and in significant relationships. Commitment to old norms and patterns must be redirected to new ones. A change in knowledge or information alone is not sufficient, although this should not necessarily be excluded. There are several common elements within this change strategy:

1. the person (e.g., patient) must be involved in working out plans of change and improvement for himself;
2. it cannot be assumed that the solution to the problem rests in acquisition of more knowledge as the problem may be in the realm of attitudes, values, and significant relationships;
3. the change agent and the person seeking change must define and solve the problem together;
4. if there are unconscious elements preventing resolution of the problem, these must be brought out;
5. the behavioral sciences provide useful concepts and methods for those seeking change.

Example

A student health professional taped an interview with a 32-year-old woman who was hospitalized for low back pain. She reviewed the tape with her instructor. The instructor noted that whenever the patient began to talk about the pain and how terrible it was, the student interrupted and changed the subject.

Discussion

The instructor identified a student behavior that needed change—the student must not interrupt a patient. She realized that the talk of pain made the student feel uncomfortable and in order to regain a sense of comfort (satisfy a need), she would interrupt and change the subject. The instructor recognized the fact that the student came from a large extended family. One of the norms within this family was that people should not complain about pain, but rather should be cheerful against all odds. The student's behavior (interrupting to prevent the patient from complaining about the pain) reflected her value system, which supported the family norm. In this situation, giving the student more information about interviewing skills was unlikely to result in changed behavior.

With these thoughts in mind, the instructor re-played the tape. This helped the student identify the problem of interrupting (THE CHANGE AGENT AND PERSON SEEKING CHANGE MUST DEFINE THE PROBLEM TOGETHER).

Instructor: Can you recall what you were feeling when you interrupted?

Student: It made me uncomfortable when she complained about the pain.

Instructor: Can you think why you might feel uncomfortable when someone complains about pain?

Student: (A long silence) I guess because no one in my family ever did. We've always been taught that the best behavior is to "grin and bear it."

The instructor had helped the student to see what caused her discomfort and her subsequent behavior of interrupting (UNCONSCIOUS ELEMENTS MUST BE BROUGHT OUT). The student's right to her own personal values was reinforced, but the instructor pointed out that adhering to this value within her professional role would prevent her from being helpful to patients experiencing pain. The instructor allowed the student time to think about this. The student returned the following week.

> *Student*: I've thought about what you said. I do want to be helpful to my patients who are in pain (COMMITMENT TO A NEW VALUE). How can I become more comfortable discussing pain?

The instructor had several ideas (USING CONCEPTS FROM THE BEHAVIORAL SCIENCES), and together they planned a series of experiences that would help the student become more comfortable discussing pain and would lead to a decrease in the interrupting behavior (THE CHANGE AGENT AND THE PERSON SEEKING CHANGE MUST SOLVE THE PROBLEM TOGETHER).

This illustrates a NORMATIVE-RE-EDUCATIVE approach to change.

3. Power-Coercive Strategies

POWER-COERCIVE strategies for change rely on the application of power in some form. Change occurs because those with less power comply with the plans, directions, and leadership of those with greater power. Rightly or wrongly, those in power are considered authorities. Political and economic sanctions may be used to effect change, or moral power may be used to play upon feelings of guilt and shame.

Example

Mr. Moffet is 56-years-old and has diabetes. He needs frequent check-ups as he is not a well-controlled diabetic, partially because he doesn't follow his treatment plan.

> *Health professional*: Well, your blood tests are not as good as I'd like to see them, but there is improvement over the last check.
>
> *Mr. Moffet*: That's good.
>
> *Health professional*: From what you say, you're sticking to your diet.
>
> *Mr. Moffet*: The wife is responsible for that.
>
> *Health professional*: Are you still drinking alcohol?
>
> *Mr. Moffet*: Yup!

Health professional:	How much?
Mr. Moffet:	Several beers during the day and a bourbon or two at night.
Health professional:	Mr. Moffet, if you don't stop drinking, I won't take care of you anymore! You're undermining the treatment plan by drinking, and you are hurting yourself . . . and your wife, I might add. She's been very concerned. (Silence) Do you understand?
Mr. Moffet:	Yeah, I understand. I'll give it a try.

Discussion

In this situation the health professional had power by virtue of knowledge and expertise in the management of diabetes. This was something the patient lacked and needed. The health professional attempted to coerce the patient into changing a habit that was dangerous to his health by threatening to withdraw his knowledge and expertise. The health professional also made Mr. Moffet feel guilty by commenting that he was hurting his wife. The health professional used a POWER–COERCIVE strategy for changing behavior.

Exercise 29:   What Strategy Was Used?

Purposes: To identify the type of strategy used to effect a change. To identify the elements of the change strategy.

Instructions: 1. Recall a situation in a health care setting where a health professional attempted to institute a change. This may have been a change in the system or a change in a patient.

2. Describe the situation. What change was proposed?

_____

_____

3. What type of change strategy (EMPIRICAL-RATIONAL, NORMATIVE-RE-EDUCATIVE, POWER-COERCIVE) was used?

_____

4.   Answer the following questions:

If the EMPIRICAL-RATIONAL approach was used:

What behavior did the change agent demonstrate that showed that he assumed that people are rational?

_____

_____

How was the change justified?

_____

_____

How would the change benefit those involved?

_____

_____

Did the change occur? _____

If the NORMATIVE-RE-EDUCATIVE approach was used:

What need was being satisfied by the behavior that was to be changed?

_____

_____

What cultural (or social) norms influenced the person(s) involved in the proposed change?

_____

_____

What value, attitude, skill, or significant relationship needed to be changed?

_____

_____

Would acquisition of new knowledge solve the problem?

_____

Did those involved in the change participate in defining the problem and working out plans for change? _____

Were there any unconscious elements that needed to be brought out? If so, what were they?

_____

_____

What methods or concepts from the behavioral sciences were used to promote the change?

_____

_____

Did the change occur? _____

If the POWER–COERCIVE approach was used:

What power did the change agent have in this situation?

_____

_____

What would the consequences have been if the change did not occur?

_____

_____

Did the change occur? _____

How did those involved in the change feel about it?

_____

_____

5. Share your responses with the rest of the group.

Questions for Discussion

- Which change strategy seems the most effective?

- What are the advantages and the disadvantages of each of the three change strategies?

F. WHAT IS A CHANGE AGENT?

A change agent is an individual, usually peripherally related to the system, who is willing to take risks to produce change. She usually relies on a strong knowledge base but is tolerant of ambiguities within the system. She has interpersonal skills that facilitate her competence. She may have another role within the system but this is usually not an administrative one.

Example

Because of budgetary constraints, there will not be staffing increases on any of the hospital wards or clinics. Despite this, patient volume is increasing. Changes will have to be made to accommodate the volume. A meeting is held to discuss this with the staff on a particular ward. The immediate reaction is resistance. The meeting continues as follows:

Jack:	Damn it. We've put hours into developing this system and getting it to work. And now they say "can" it. Well no way . . . .
Liz:	I agree. Why should we change it? Let's tell them no.
Sara (unit director):	I recognize you're upset . . . but we can't continue the way we are!!
Mary:	Sara, what are the reasons for the problems?
Sara:	The government says health care is becoming too expensive. There is just no money in the pot.
Mary:	And has administration told us how we must accommodate the constraints—or can we submit suggestions?
Liz:	Maybe we should decrease the teaching . . . .
Leanne:	Or maybe we could deal with some of the problems in groups rather than individually.

Mary: Maybe we should make a list of priorities so
that we can relinquish the tasks we know are
less important but retain the ones that are?

It was obvious at the onset of the meeting that changes were
going to occur. The staff, however, needed time to protest and
voice their concerns about the loss of something they had worked
hard to develop. In other words, they resisted. The unit director,
recognizing the upset and RESISTANCE, labelled it. It was the job
of the CHANGE AGENT, Mary, to readdress why change was
being "ordered," and question the way change was to be implemented. Once she had established an outlet for the group's energy,
the individuals in the group were able to begin redirecting themselves. Mary did not suggest the change, she merely rerouted the
group's energy into a very change-directed pattern.

All organizations, groups, and teams are influenced by change,
whether it originates from within or from outside. Even resistance
where none existed before is a change. The role of a change agent
is to facilitate the ease with which the change occurs.

Sometimes, when a team is having interpersonal difficulties,
a change consultant may be requested. This request may be internally or externally initiated and is more likely to be successful
if internally requested.

The consultant is introduced from outside the team and is
usually skilled at problem-solving. He would encourage the team
to self-diagnose difficulties and aid them in solving their own problems. His objectivity would usually enable him to spot trouble
areas, and he could then reveal these to the group. He would
facilitate the group working together.

G. BEHAVIOR CHANGE
TECHNIQUES

Altering behavior can occur at a personal or interpersonal level.
There may be an aspect of our own behavior which is proving a
disadvantage and which we'd like to change (e.g., nail-biting or
aggressive behavior). As health professionals interacting with patients and peers, we frequently encounter behaviors in others
which prevent them from having successful social interactions. We
may be formally assigned responsibility for altering this behavior
(e.g., with patients) or may accept informal responsibility with a
peer to help him change his behavior. Techniques derived from
behavior modification have been successful in changing behavior.

1. Behavior Modification

Behavior modification is based on the theory that all behaviors are maintained by their consequences or outcome. When you perceive the outcomes of your behavior as having a payoff for yourself, you are more likely to repeat the behavior. When there are no desirable consequences for your behavior, you are unlikely to repeat it.

Example

4-year-old Mary is seen with her parents at the Child and Family Clinic because of behavioral problems. The child has been biting and spitting at adults, her parents, and older siblings. The nursery school Mary attends has had no difficulty with her.

During the interview, while the therapist was talking with Mary's parents, Mary began to pull her father's hair. Her father responded as follows:

Father: Mary stop that!

Mary: (Pulls harder.)

Father: Mary stop that or I'll get angry.

Mary: (Continues to pull hair.)

Father: (Shrugs his shoulders and begins to play with the child.)

Mary's behavior, though we might call it undesirable, was earning her a fair amount of attention. Father may have been annoyed, but eventually he stopped talking with his wife and the health professional and devoted his attention to Mary. Mary was able to distract her father, gain his attention, and take "the heat off" discussions about her behavior. Her father unwittingly encouraged her in her hair pulling antics by paying attention to her misbehavior.

The therapist intervened in the following manner:

Therapist to Mr. Jones: I think Mary is uncomfortable. She doesn't like what we're discussing, and she's not getting much attention right now. (LABELLING and OFFERING ALTERNATIVE PLAN)

Therapist to Mary:	Mary, I know you don't like what we are talking about, but it is important. You can talk with us about this or play with the toys in the corner. Biting, spitting, and kicking are not allowed in this room. If you continue to bite, spit, or kick you will have to sit by yourself in a quiet room. (This technique is familiar to Mary since the nursery school uses it.)
Therapist to Parents:	How do you usually handle it when Mary doesn't follow through?

The therapist has taken control of the situation. She has labelled the undesirable behavior and the reasons why it was occurring. She has offered behavioral alternatives, which are acceptable, but also offered consequences if the undesirable behavior recurs. When behavior change is being attempted, there is often resistance to this change. It is important that Mary know the consequence of her behavior since the behavior was very difficult to ignore when it occurred.

Several minutes later, Mary, who had been sitting quietly up to this point, gets off her chair. She approaches the therapist and kicks her in the shin. The therapist quietly gets up, takes the child by the hand, and leads her out of the room to an adjoining unoccupied one. She tells Mary she must stay there for five minutes and then can rejoin the family. Mrs. Brown, who is working in the corridor, will tell Mary when the time is up. Five minutes later, the child sheepishly enters the room. She goes quietly to the play area, where she stays until the interview ends. The therapist congratulates her several times for the desired behavior.

The kicking might not have occurred if the therapist had reinforced Mary's quiet behavior at the beginning. However, this did not occur, and once Mary had misbehaved, it was important that the therapist follow through. Providing Mary with "TIME OUT" allowed the interview to continue. "Time out" deliberately placed Mary in a safe, isolated situation where her angry behavior had no victims. It was an obvious way of ignoring her and providing no audience for aggressive acts on her part. Mary was not only isolated and ignored, she was also aware that fun and exciting things were available in an area she had lost access to. Time out also allowed the therapist a chance to "model" behavior modification for the parents.

Behavior modification uses two basic techniques: IGNORING and REINFORCING. Ignoring occurs when you pay no attention to the undesirable behavior you want to eliminate in someone else. Reinforcement is the method of rewarding someone for desired behavior. In the above example, the therapist ignored Mary's acting out behavior and reinforced her desirable behavior. Systematic ignoring of undesirable behavior over a period of time results in less frequent occurrence of the behavior. Reinforcement of desired behavior when performed systematically leads to more frequent occurrence of that behavior. By ignoring Mary's aggressive behavior (biting, spitting, and kicking) and reinforcing her positive behavior (playing with toys), the therapist was able to modify Mary's behavior. The parents, following through on the same approach, were able to develop more assertive, cooperative behavior and diminish the aggressive, negative behavior.

Example

John, a psychiatric patient, had been regularly ripping up the magazines and newspapers on the ward. This produced a negative reaction on the part of other patients who enjoyed the reading material. They became very upset and angry with John. The health care team involved had documented the frequency with which this behavior was occurring. They decided to initiate a behavior modification program. John's undesirable behavior was to be ignored by the staff and other patients. John would be awarded a "coin" for each third of the day he could get through without tearing up a magazine or newspaper. These "coins" could be exchanged for privileges. John was particularly anxious to get access to the billiard table, and this was a possibility if he had five "coins." The other patients received similar rewards when they were able to cooperate with the behavior desired from them (i.e., ignoring John's aggressive behavior).

There was an immediate decrease in John's magazine ripping, but shortly thereafter, he started it again. Other patients and staff ignored him so that the attention he had previously gotten for the same behavior was not forthcoming. The staff quickly reinforced him by praising him when he was not ripping up magazines.

Tangible rewards came frequently, and he was soon playing billiards regularly.

Rewards can be intrinsic or extrinsic. In behavior modification, tangible extrinsic rewards (e.g., candy, tokens) or social rewards like praise are most successful. As time passes, we incorporate the good feelings produced by rewards and are content to strive only for these intrinsic rewards. But a reward that is reinforcing must always be offered to the person you are trying to help change if change is to occur. Changing the strength or presence of the reinforcer changes the behavior.

Some more examples are shown in the following table:

Behavior	Consequence	Effects of Consequence on Behavior	Conclusion
1. You do someone a favor.	He thanks you and on another occasion does you a favor.	You, in future, do other favors for him.	The positive consequence has reinforced your behavior.
2. You do someone a favor.	He doesn't thank you, nor does he do you any favors.	You don't do him any more favors.	The negative consequence doesn't reinforce your behavior.
3. Mary pulls her father's hair.	Her father yells at her.	Mary continues to pull her father's hair.	"Being yelled at" is a form of behavior Mary likes. Bugging her father is a reinforcer to her.
4. Mary pulls her father's hair.	Her father ignores her.	Mary stops pulling her father's hair.	Mary's misbehavior is no longer being reinforced by her father's attention.

There are certain rules that should be followed to make behavior modification effective and thus eliminate another person's negative behavior.

1. Identify specifically the undesirable behavior you want stopped (e.g., biting, spitting, tearing up magazines).

2. Identify specifically the desired behavior you want started (e.g., playing with toys, leaving magazines alone).

3. Identify reinforcers you can use to reinforce desirable behavior and thus increase its frequency. Offering chocolate ice cream to a chocolate ice cream hater is no reward.

4. Chart the frequency of the undesired behavior for a period prior to commencing the program. Continue to graph during the program in order to evaluate the program.

5. Begin the program. Tell the other person what you expect and what the reward will be. (For example, "I would like you to sit quietly and play with your dolls. If you do so, your mother and father and I will be very pleased, we can finish soon, and you can go home.") The person should be aware of the reinforcers, when they will come, and what they will be. There must also be a consistent approach by all those involved (i.e., the undesirable behavior must be IGNORED every time and the desirable behavior REINFORCED every time). If the other patients had not been involved in John's program, their angry reaction might have been sufficient reinforcement to maintain his behavior despite staff efforts to eliminate it.

    If you find yourself getting angry at the other person's undesirable behavior, leave his presence rather than reinforce him with your angry reaction. By assertively withdrawing from the situation you are still able to ignore the behavior and remain assertive.

6. Continue the program for a time, monitoring it carefully. If the expected change is not occurring, then you are probably not IGNORING and REINFORCING properly. Are you consistently and completely ignoring the negative behavior? Are you consistently rewarding the other person with a reward he really wants?

7. If the desired changes are occurring—congratulations! But you're not through yet. Continue to ignore the undesired behavior and gradually make the reinforcer more difficult to obtain (so that even better performance is required for pay-offs). Begin intermittent reinforcement (reinforce occasionally instead of every time).

8. Continue the program until the undesired behavior is eliminated and the desired behavior is based on social or intrinsic rewards.

Exercise 30: Designing a Behavior Modification Program

Purpose: To practice designing a behavior modification program.

Instructions: 1. Divide the group into pairs.

2. Using the situation described below, develop with your partner a behavior modification program to modify the personal hygiene habits of staff on the ward described below.

Situation

A new unit director has been hired to coordinate the care on a surgical unit. She is disturbed by the appearance of the staff on the ward and its implications for aseptic technique. There is a uniform policy at the hospital, which is not enforced. Rather than alienate the staff by enforcing the policy, she decides to use a behavior modification program. Her first goal is to have staff members' long hair out of the way of sterile open dressing trays.

Instructions: 1. Divide the group into pairs.

2. Using the situation described below, develop with your partner a behavior modification program to modify the personal hygiene habits of staff on this ward.

3. Identify the undesirable behavior in this situation.

_____

_____

4. Identify the desired behavior in this situation.

_____

_____

5. Identify some potential reinforcers the unit director could use to reinforce the desired behavior.

_____

_____

6. Describe how you would implement your behavior modification program using your reinforcers.

_____

_____

_____

_____

7. Have each pair describe their behavior modification program to the group.

Questions for Discussion

- Did everyone agree on what the desirable and undesirable behaviors were?
- What reinforcers were seen as most rewarding for the staff?

Exercise 31: Designing Your Own Behavior Modification Program

Purpose: To design a behavior modification program to modify another person's behavior.

Instructions: 1. Identify someone whose behavior you would like to help change. This person could be a patient, a health professional, or just someone you know. Briefly describe the behavior you want to change.

_____

_____

_____

2. Identify the desirable behavior that you would like (or this person would like) to see occur more frequently.

_____

_____

_____

3. Identify some reinforcers you could use to reward the desirable behavior.

_____

_____

_____

4. Describe the steps you would follow to implement your behavior program. How will you ignore the undesirable behavior? How often will you reward the desirable behavior?

_____

_____

_____

_____

_____

5. Divide the group into pairs. Together with your partner, take turns discussing your behavior modification programs.

Questions for Discussion

- Was the undesirable behavior described in specific terms? (For example, "He frequently criticizes the way I dress" is specific; "He is mean to me" is not.)

- Was the desirable behavior described in specific terms? ("I want her to pay attention and look at me when I talk to her" is specific; "I want her to be nice to me" is not.)

- If you were to try your program out and it didn't work, what might be some reasons it didn't work?

SUMMARY

A health professional needs the ability to adapt to change. He also needs to be able to motivate others to change. A knowledge of change, change theory, change agents, and change methodology, such as behavior modification, is necessary if these aspects of practice are to be accomplished.

6
Developing Assertion Skills

A. WHAT IS ASSERTION?

Frequently, as a health professional, you will be expected to express an opinion and take responsibility for your own actions. Assertion, or assertive behavior, involves standing up for your legitimate rights without violating the rights of others or having bad feelings in the process.

But how do you directly express your own feelings, preferences, needs, or opinions in a manner that is neither threatening, nor punishing to another person?

Example

Five-year-old Peter has a blood disorder that requires chemotherapy. Before receiving his medication at the clinic visit, he must have blood taken. It is an important and necessary function in his assessment and treatment.

Previously, Peter has been distressed and cried about the procedure. Today, however, he is angry and very frightened. He screams, clings to his mother, and hits out at the health professional responsible for drawing his blood.

Non-Assertive Response.

Health professional: Uhhh . . . well . . . It's okay, Peter. Maybe we won't have to take blood today. Maybe . . .

Aggressive Response.

Health professional: Go ahead. Scream all you want, BUT I'm going to take blood . . . even if it takes me five stabs, and if *I* don't get it, somebody else will.

Assertive Response.

Health professional: Peter, I know that you're scared and that you don't like this, but it's important to help you feel well. I'll be really fast, and you can help by holding on tight to Mommy. Mommy, have you got the bandaid ready?

Peter, who stimulated all three responses, was actually being quite outspoken, in a way that most 5-year-olds, faced with a threatening and anxiety-provoking situation, can be.

The NON-ASSERTIVE response, in this instance, could have a very destructive result. The health professional, in order to appease the child, suggested something that both she and Peter's mother knew was impossible if treatment were to be constructively and safely provided. She also reinforced Peter's misbehavior by giving in to his tantrum. Having gotten his way this time, it is likely that Peter will protest similarly in the future. A non-assertive response is a hesitant, conciliatory way of behaving in which true feelings are never revealed. Non-assertive behaviors include: self-denial, self-depreciation, inhibition, and bending over backwards to please others.

The AGGRESSIVE response was one that put the child down and denied him his right to protest. The health professional didn't allow him any bodily control over his actions. Peter's mother may see his prognosis and treatment as functions of the health professional's perception of the kind of child Peter is. If she can't control her son's behavior, will they think he is worthy of treatment?

The aggressive response was very self-expressive and self-indulgent. Unfortunately, it occurred at Peter's expense. In fact, the health professional made a decision for Peter, further exaggerating the lack of control that he felt.

The ASSERTIVE response produced positive results. The child, though still somewhat tearful, willingly participated and proudly displayed his bandaid to the clinic personnel. The health professional had shown understanding for Peter's behavior while positively giving him the message that the procedure would be done. She thus avoided the dilemma of letting Peter choose, only to be over-ruled. This alleviated any guilt Peter or his mother might feel about exposing him to the venipuncture. The assertive response is an open, direct, self-enhancing way of expressing personal feelings and opinions.

Assertion can also be looked at in win-lose terms. Using the previous example where Peter is having blood drawn against his better wishes, we can see the following behaviors:

Non-Assertive Response. When the health professional responded non-assertively to Peter, she did not accomplish her task, which was to draw blood from Peter. Therefore, Peter won (he wasn't poked) and the health professional lost (she didn't do her job and felt badly). This is summarized in the diagram below:

		Outcome
Peter's behavior:	Unintentionally AGGRESSIVE	WIN
Health Professional's Response:	NON-ASSERTIVE	LOSE
Task:	Not accomplished	

Aggressive Response. In this situation, the health professional responded with anger and aggression towards the child. This produced even more anger from Peter and probably prevented the task being accomplished. Thus, the health professional felt better (won) for having vented her anger, but the child lost even more control of his anger.

		Outcome
Peter's behavior:	Unintentionally AGGRESSIVE	LOSE
Health Professional's Response	AGGRESSIVE	WIN
Task:	Accomplished at Peter's expense or not accomplished because of Peter's non-participation.	

Assertive Response. In this situation, the health professional showed respect for Peter's feelings. She was in control of herself, and she allowed Peter responsibility for himself. The task was accomplished. This was a "win" solution for everyone.

		Outcome
Peter's behavior:	Unintentionally AGGRESSIVE	WIN
Health Professional's Response:	ASSERTIVE	WIN
Task:	Accomplished	

Assertive behavior allows everyone involved the opportunity to benefit to some degree. The health professional doesn't take responsibility for anyone's feelings other than her own.

The table below shows the kind of verbal and non-verbal behaviors used by non-assertive, aggressive, and assertive individuals.

EXAMPLES OF ASSERTIVE, AGGRESSIVE, AND
NON-ASSERTIVE BEHAVIOR

Behaviors	Non-Assertive	Aggressive	Assertive
Verbal	apologetic words, hedging, rambling, failing to say what is meant	loaded words, accusations, vague, superior, haughty words, "you" messages that label the other person	statement of wants, objective words, "I" messages, honest statement of feelings
Non-verbal General	actions instead of words (you don't say what you feel) looking as though you don't mean what you say	flippant, sarcastic style, air of superiority	confident, congruent messages
Specific Voice	weak, distant, soft, wavering	tense, shrill, loud, cold, deadly quiet, demanding, superior, authoritarian	firm, warm, confident
Eyes	averted, downcast, teary, pleading	expressionless, cold, narrowed, staring	warm, frank
Stance	stooped, excessive leaning for support	hands on hips, feet apart	relaxed
Hands	fidgety, clammy	abrupt gestures, fists pounding or clenched	gestures at appropriate times

Exercise 32:   Getting To Know the Non-Assertive You

Purpose: To identify non-assertive behavior. To identify some advantages and disadvantages of your non-assertive behavior.

Instructions: 1. Think of an occasion when you were non-assertive (submissive) in your relationship with

another person (e.g., a patient or health professional). Briefly describe the incident.

_____

_____

_____

_____

_____

_____

_____

2. What feelings did you have as a result of these
   incidents (e.g., sad, depressed, angry, furious,
   anxious, etc.)?

_____

_____

3. Use the space below to show the ways you and
   the other person won and/or lost.

In what ways did you: Win _____

                         Lose _____

In what ways did the
   other person: Win _____

                         Lose _____

4. Share this in pairs.

Exercise 33:   Getting To Know the Aggressive You

Purpose: To identify your aggressive behavior. To identify
              some advantages and disadvantages of your aggres-
              sive behavior.

Instructions: 1. Think of an occasion when you were aggressive
                     in your relationship with another person (e.g.,

a patient or health professional). Briefly describe the incident. _____

_____

_____

_____

_____

_____

_____

2. What feelings did you have as a result of this situation (e.g., sad, depressed, angry, furious, anxious, etc.)?

_____

_____

3. Use the space below to show the ways you and the other person won and/or lost.

In what ways did you: Win _____

                          Lose _____

In what ways did the
    other person: Win _____

                          Lose _____

4. Share this in pairs.

Exercise 34:   Getting To Know the Assertive You

Purpose: To identify your assertive behavior. To identify some advantages and disadvantages of your assertive behavior.

Instructions: 1. Think of a time when you were assertive in your relationship with another person (e.g., a

patient or health professional). Briefly describe
the incident. _____

_____

_____

_____

_____

_____

_____

2. What feelings did you have as a result of this
    situation (e.g., sad, depressed, angry, furious,
    anxious, etc.)?

_____

_____

3. Use the space below to show the ways you and
    the other person won and/or lost.

In what ways did you: Win _____

                           Lose _____

In what ways did the
    other person: Win _____

                           Lose _____

4. Share this in pairs.

B. TYPES OF ASSERTION SKILLS

There are several categories of assertive behavior that you can use
to express yourself in different situations. They are:

1. Being Confrontive
2. Saying No
3. Making Requests
4. Expressing Opinions
5. Initiating Conversations

6. Self-disclosing

7. Expressing Affection

The first two categories are related to constructive expression of negative feelings, such as anger or dissatisfaction.

1.   Being Confrontive

Example

A health professional learner had requested permission to attend an epilepsy clinic. A contract had been devised in which the learner's needs were identified, the kind of patients he would best gain by seeing were determined, and the particular dates of attendance stated. He was to let the team leader know in advance if he were unable to be present, since there was a long list of learners anxious to attend this particular clinic. On the designated day, the patients arrived, but the student did not, nor did he send any message. Both patients and staff were inconvenienced. The student phoned the next morning and said, "Sorry, I forgot. But I'll be there next Tuesday." How would you respond if you were the team leader?

Non-Assertive Response: "Uh . . . Oh sure . . . See you then . . .!"

The learner violated the original contract despite your having completed your part of the bargain. What is to prevent him doing it again? And how did you deal with the anger you felt towards this student who frustrated and overworked you and your team members? Why do you give the impression that it's reasonable to let you down?

Aggressive Response: "And just WHO do you think you are? You've blown it. You've got your nerve thinking you can just come when you please!"

You dealt with your anger and in the process you put the student down. But what if he had a plausible excuse? You'll never hear it now, and you've gained a reputation as the clinician to avoid because of your temper!

Assertive Response: "We had a contract. You agreed to let me know in advance if you were unable to attend the clinic. Because you didn't call me, another person missed a chance to take your place. I am disappointed about this.''

You have confronted the learner with the fact that your rights were violated. You have released your anger constructively and yet maintained your relationship with the student. If he has a plausible explanation, he can offer it now. Otherwise, he can consider the contract broken.

BEING CONFRONTIVE means defining when you've been hurt, but doing so without being aggressive to the other person.

2. Saying No

Example

A recently hired health professional was previously employed in a community setting. In that position, she was not expected to administer medication intramuscularly, and her skills have become rusty. She is now in a situation where injections will be frequently ordered. Today she approaches you and says, "This patient has an I.M. ordered. I wonder if you'd mind giving it?"

Non-Assertive Response: "Ummm . . . Yeah . . . Okay. Sure. That's okay . . ."

Although you're saying yes, you really want to say no. Are you saying yes because you're afraid she'll be angry with you if you say no? But how many I.M.'s will you have to give for her?

Aggressive Response: "Look, it's your patient. Why did you take the job if you don't know how to do the work? Do it yourself."

You've labelled her professionally incompetent, and if she follows your suggestion, you may have caused a dangerous situation for the patient.

Assertive Response: "No, I won't give it because I think you're able. Would it help if we reviewed the technique and I went with you while you gave it?"

You were able to say no politely, and yet aid your colleague, thereby ensuring the patient's safety.

SAYING NO means declining the other person's unreasonable request without putting the other person down.

MAKING REQUESTS and EXPRESSING OPINIONS are assertion skills that apply especially to emotionally neutral situations where requests, suggestions, opinions, and information are dispensed and solicited.

3. Making Requests

Example

You are a health professional working afternoons on a surgical ward. Your case assignment is heavy, and you are becoming aware of changes in the status of a fresh post-op patient. You know this will require your spending much more time with him, monitoring his vital signs and general status. You are going to need some help.

Non-Assertive Response: "Gee, I'm tired, and my back hurts . . . boy, will I be glad when this shift is over."

This response gives unclear, indirect messages, which are difficult for others to interpret. As a result, there may be no offer of help, and patients may suffer.

Aggressive Response: "Damn it! Can't any of you see that I need help? This patient's in trouble and you don't even care."

This response is accusing and hurtful. You may get the help you need, but not willingly.

Assertive Response: You say to the team leader: "Mr. Jones' status has changed, and I'll have to spend more time with him. Could we redistribute the patient assignment, so that I can?"

This response was a clear message and given to the appropriate person. She can redistribute the patient assignment and get the added resources to deal with the ill patient.

MAKING REQUESTS means asking someone to do something for you.

4. Expressing Opinions

Example

A day care surgical program is being proposed for the hospital in which you work. You previously were involved in organizing and running a very successful unit at another hospital. You have been invited to a planning

session, and the chairperson has asked for your opinion
of the submitted ideas.

Non-Assertive Response: "Uh . . . Gee . . . It all sounds really
fine . . . Just great . . . ."
Your response was so ambivalent that it contributes nothing.
Mistakes that you learned to avoid through experience may be
made by the planning committee. You have missed a chance to
help them learn from your practical experience.

Aggressive Response: "You are completely off course. It won't
work the way you're planning it. I'll show you what to do."
By taking over, you may alienate the other committee members, who may have some good ideas. They may discontinue their
committee membership or yours.

Assertive Response: "I think suggestions 1, 3, and 7 are very
workable for these reasons . . . However, I wonder if everyone is
really clear about the program objectives? That was the biggest
problem we faced at . . . hospital."
By answering the question clearly and directly, based on your
own experience, you are being assertive.
EXPRESSING OPINIONS means sharing your beliefs and
ideas with others.

5.   Initiating Conversations

Example

You are attending a behavioral science seminar and
recognize that a fellow participant is a member of a
community agency that you would like to know more
about. The morning coffee break is coming up.

Non-Assertive Response: You think to yourself, "Should I
ask her if we can meet over coffee? Oh, she's probably got other
plans. I wonder where the washroom is?"
By remaining silent because you fear rejection, you miss
an opportunity to meet someone and get to know about her
agency.

Aggressive Response: "I want to talk to you. What's your
agency's philosophy on . . .?"

By overwhelming the other person and forcing her to take a stand immediately, you may intimidate her and end abruptly what could have been a fruitful conversation.

Assertive Response: "Hi. My name is Janet. I work for the local health agency. I was interested in some of your comments and wondered if they reflected the thinking of your agency?"

By initiating the interaction in a warm, tactful manner and showing a genuine interest in the other individual, you are being assertive.

INITIATING CONVERSATIONS means approaching someone you are interested in meeting and initiating a conversation.

6. Self-Disclosing

INITIATING CONVERSATIONS, SELF-DISCLOSING and EXPRESSING AFFECTION relate to the expression of positive emotions like interest in others, caring, loving, affection, and trust.

Example

A fellow health professional seems distracted and distressed at work. She fumbles tasks she usually handles with competence. You ask her if anything is wrong.

Non-Assertive Response: "No, nothing. . . I'm fine. Pass me that book, please."

The health professional, by withholding information that is obviously distressing her has missed an opportunity for some help which might have been forthcoming. If she continues to fumble her work, having said all was well, she may antagonize some of her peers.

Aggressive Response: "Look, leave me alone. I'm absolutely fine. Haven't you anything better to do than bother me?"

An aggressive response of this nature could antagonize the caring enquirer. The result is that the person in difficulty doesn't get the support she needs.

Assertive Response: "I feel all thumbs today. Guess I'm having trouble concentrating. My father was taken to the hospital last night with chest pain, and I'm really worried."

This individual is not incapacitated by her own distress. She recognizes her own response as a natural one and by sharing its cause, is able to receive support from her peer.

SELF-DISCLOSING means sharing intimate experiences and feelings with others.

7.   Expressing Affection

Example

You work in a cystic fibrosis unit and the chronicity of the disease means you know most of the patients well. At this time, two of the teenagers are in particular difficulty with their disease and you are working closely with them. One of your colleagues approaches you and states how impressed she is with your skills in working with this age group. You answer:

Non-Assertive Response: "Uhh . . . Mmmm . . . Are you going out for lunch?"

Someone complimenting your skills is really complimenting you. The non-assertive individual has difficulty receiving and responding to a compliment of this nature.

Aggressive Response: "Well, of course, I'm good. I've had years of experience."

Making a joke of an intimate compliment is an act of aggression towards the person giving you the compliment. Compliments may not be so frequently forthcoming in the future.

Assertive Response: "Thank you. I've been at it for awhile and experience teaches many lessons. That doesn't mean it's easy through. I appreciate the compliment."

The assertive person can accept compliments and give them. He is a caring friend.

EXPRESSING AFFECTION means sharing with another person your liking and caring for him.

All of the previously mentioned assertion skills are summarized in the table on page 195 which shows the typical kind of emotion involved with each of the assertion skills.

ASSERTION SKILL ————►EXPRESSES ————► TYPICAL EMOTION

1. BEING CONFRONTIVE 2. SAYING NO	Negative Emotions
3. MAKING REQUESTS 4. EXPRESSING OPINIONS	Emotionally Neutral
5. INITIATING CONVERSATIONS 6. SELF-DISCLOSING 7. EXPRESSING AFFECTION	Positive Emotions

Exercise 35:   Identifying Your Own Assertion Skills

Purpose: To identify your own assertion skills.

Instructions: 1.   The group leader writes the seven assertion categories on a chalkboard and puts a checkmark (✓) beside the two assertion skills he feels weakest at. The rest of the group is then invited to come up to the chalkboard to check off their two weakest assertion skills. The result is a profile of the groups weakest (and strongest) assertion skills.

2.   Divide the class into small groups. Each group agrees on which assertion skill is the most important and which assertion skill is the least important for health professionals to have. The seven assertion skills should be ranked in order of importance (1 = most important, 7 = least important). As your group decides on the rank order of each assertion skill, write down the rank assigned to each assertion skill in the space provided below:

RANK	*ASSERTION SKILL*
_____	BEING CONFRONTIVE
_____	SAYING NO
_____	MAKING REQUESTS
_____	EXPRESSING OPINIONS
_____	INITIATING CONVERSATIONS
_____	SELF-DISCLOSING
_____	EXPRESSING AFFECTION

3. The group leader next writes on a chalkboard the ranks assigned to each assertion skill by the small groups. Each small group should state why it feels the assertion skill it ranked as "1" deserves the rank of "1". The leader should total up the ranks assigned to each skill. The skill with the lowest total is the assertion skill rated as most important by the entire class.

Questions for Discussion:

- Which assertion skill was rated as most important by the group as a whole? Least important?
- Which assertion skills—those dealing with expression of negative feelings (Being Confrontive and Saying No); those dealing with task situations (Making Requests, and Expressing Opinions); or those dealing with expressions of positive feelings (Initiating Conversations, Self-Disclosing and Expressing Affection)—were seen as most important for health professionals to have?

Assertion is a synonym for personal competence. Being assertive means being constructively effective with your patients and with other health professionals. Being assertive means expressing constructively your positive, as well as your negative, emotions.

A number of studies have shown that health professionals have difficulty handling aggressive patients and aggressive health professionals. Because health professionals seem to have more difficulty in asserting themselves in conflict situations, the rest of this chapter will focus on the assertion skills for handling aggression.

C. DEVELOPING CONFRONTATION SKILLS

CONFRONTATION is the assertive skill of pointing out to someone his aggressive behavior. CONFRONTATION skills are useful to halt another person's aggressive behavior towards yourself by alerting him that you will not tolerate such behavior. There are three main CONFRONTATION skills:

1. "I"CONFRONTATION
2. DESC CONFRONTATION
3. DISC CONFRONTATION

1.   "I" Confrontation

Example

A health professional tutorial group has decided to examine the implications of the environment of pregnancy. You and another student, Jim, volunteer to prepare data on smoking and its correlation with prematurity. You divide the task and arrange to meet in order to assimilate the data for the large group. You have spent several hours in preparation time and arrive at the meeting eager for action. You find that Jim has done nothing. You decide to confront him.

You: Damn it. That's not fair. You never carry your share. Your word's worthless. Why don't you get your act together. We're all fed up with doing all the work. ("You" CONFRONTATION)

Jim: Have you finished? Just who do you think you are? (AGGRESSIVE response)

When you are angry or frustrated, it is easy to explode with generalizations and sweeping criticism (e.g., "You never carry your share."). Usually though, the directed anger hurts the other person and forces reciprocal anger of equal or greater dimensions (e.g., "Just who do you think you are?").

An angry, accusing, and attacking confrontation directed at the other person is called a "You" Confrontation, or a "You are" Confrontation. A "You are" Confrontation (i.e., a "Here's what's wrong with you" confrontation) blocks constructive communication and produces a defensive reaction in the other person.

The situation can be dealt with in a way that is not blaming or attacking. This requires, however some objectivity so that the situation is seen and described factually. It also requires that the confronting data contain your feelings and that you not assume the offender's supposed motives. This type of confrontation is called an "I" CONFRONTATION.

You: When you agree to help me with the prematurity part of the tutorial and then you don't come prepared, I feel annoyed because it means we have to hold an additional meeting that wastes my time. ("I" CONFRONTATION)

Jim: You're right. I should have had the work done. I'm sorry. How would it be if I coordinate the data? (ASSERTIVE response)

An "I" CONFRONTATION (i.e., "This is how I am feeling about your behavior" CONFRONTATION) facilitates constructive communication.

"You" CONFRONTATION = AGGRESSION
"I" CONFRONTATION = ASSERTION

An "I" CONFRONTATION has three components:

A BEHAVIOR DESCRIPTION,

A statement of NEGATIVE CONSEQUENCE,

And a FEELING DESCRIPTION.

When you make an "I" CONFRONTATION, you calmly describe the actual aggressive behavior that occurred (BEHAVIOR DESCRIPTION) and your feelings in response to the aggressive behavior (FEELING DESCRIPTION). In addition, you can describe the negative consequence of the aggressive behavior on you (NEGATIVE CONSEQUENCE). This negative consequence is in fact the reason why you are complaining, and it is also the obvious reason why there should be a change in the other person's behavior. When you are learning to make an "I" CONFRONTATION, you may find it helpful to make the following responses:

"When you . . ." (State your BEHAVIOR DESCRIPTION)
"I feel . . ." (State your FEELING DESCRIPTION)
"Because . . ." (State the NEGATIVE CONSEQUENCE for you)

Example

"When *you* agree to help with the prematurity part of of the tutorial and then don't come prepared (BEHAVIOR DESCRIPTION) *I feel* annoyed (FEELING DESCRIPTION) *because* it means we have to hold an additional meeting, and that wastes my time (NEGATIVE CONSEQUENCE)."

Summary

$$\begin{array}{c}\text{Behavior} \\ \text{Description}\end{array} + \begin{array}{c}\text{Feeling} \\ \text{Description}\end{array} + \begin{array}{c}\text{Negative} \\ \text{Consequence}\end{array} = \text{"I" Confrontation}$$

However, in using "I" CONFRONTATION, it is important to remember two important points. Use "I" CONFRONTATION only with persons you care about and who care about you. Do not use "I" CONFRONTATION with people who don't care about your feelings, people who manipulate you, or people who deliberately try to hurt you. People who care about you will be responsive to your feelings. Sharing your feelings about things that are annoying or concerning you will be more likely to elicit change.

People who have no special relationship with you however, have no vested interest in making you feel good. In fact, sharing your feelings may provide them with ammunition to meet their own needs at your expense. So, use "I" CONFRONTATION carefully.

Exercise 36:   Writing "I" Confrontations

Purpose: To practice writing complete "I" CONFRONTATIONS.

Instructions: 1.   Divide the class into pairs.

2.   Together with your partner, write a destructive "You" CONFRONTATION and a constructive "I" CONFRONTATION for one situation shown below.

3.   Role play "You" CONFRONTATION and your "I" CONFRONTATION for the rest of the group.

Situation	*"YOU"* *CONFRONTATION*	*"I"* *CONFRONTATION*
1. One of the main team members is chronically late for clinic. You can't start without him. Today he arrives one hour late.	_____	_____
2. You are lined up at the coffeeshop during your break and someone steps ahead of you.	_____	_____
3. When the patient in room 21 wants help, he keeps shouting for you instead of using his buzzer.	_____	_____

4. Your friend Alice is   _____ _____
   constantly criticizing the
   way you dress. Today she   _____ _____
   says to you, "Gosh, are
   you wearing those old   _____ _____
   shoes again?"

                                        _____ _____

Questions for Discussion

- How did you feel when faced by a "You" CONFRON-
  TATION?
- Was there a difference when you faced the "I" CON-
  FRONTATION?

2. DESC Confrontation

When a more detailed confrontation, one which clearly defines
how you want the other person to change, is required, you can use
a DESC CONFRONTATION (Bower and Bower, 1976). DESC is
an acronym, each letter representing a critical word (D—Describe,
E — Express, S — Specify, C — Consequences). In fact, it is an "I"
CONFRONTATION with an accompanying request.

Example

Because of dramatic increases in patient volume in the
hospital emergency department, there must be a redistribution of roles of the health professionals working
there. A compulsory meeting is held in order to determine the best way of facilitating this change. The one
health professional who is most resistant to the change,
Joan, is notable by her absence from this meeting. As
unit director, you decide to deal with the situation by
making a DESC CONFRONTATION to Joan.

Describe: A compulsory staff meeting was held yesterday
             to examine role redistribution. You were not there.

Express: I was annoyed because we had difficulty getting
             group consensus about the changes the department is
             having to undergo to provide competent care.

Specify: I'd like you to be present at the next meeting and
             participate as best you can.

Consequences (Positive):   If you do so, I and the rest of the staff will appreciate it. (*Negative*): If not, we will have to question your commitment to increasing patient care.

A DESC CONFRONTATION contains the following components:

1. It describes the other person's behavior.
2. It expresses your feelings about the situation.
3. It specifies that you want the other person to do to improve the situation.
4. It expresses consequences:
    (a) Positive—it points out to the other person the positive result of his complying with your request;
    (b) Negative—if he refuses or seems likely to refuse, it points out the negative results that will occur if he does not comply with your request.

Note: Avoid negative consequences unless absolutely necessary as it may provoke aggression in the other person. If you do use a negative consequence, however, relate the consequence logically to the other person's irresponsible behavior. Also, give the other person the opportunity to respond by asking, "Will you do that?" after your "specify" statement.

Exercise 37:   Writing a DESC Confrontation

Purpose: To practice writing a DESC CONFRONTATION

Instructions: In pairs, write a DESC CONFRONTATION for the situation below.

Situation
You share an office with a colleague. He is an "accumulator," and the office is rapidly filling with boxes and loose papers. There is no rhyme or reason to their placement, and the office is beginning to look like a disaster area. You must interview in this room, and you resent the mess. You decide to ask him to clean it up.

Describe: _____

_____

_____

Express: _____

_____

_____

Specify: _____

_____

_____

Consequences:
(Positive)   _____

_____

(Negative)   _____

_____

Have several pairs role-play their DESC CONFRONTATION for the group.

3. DISC Confrontation

A DISC CONFRONTATION is similar to a DESC CONFRONTA-TION but is used when confronting someone who may not care about your feelings. With this sort of person you omit an expression of your feelings. Sharing feelings may not always be appropriate, in fact it may be detrimental to the desired outcome, especially if the aggressive individual uses your feelings against you. On these occasions an appropriate choice is a DISC CONFRONTA-TION (DISC is an acronym for D — Describe, I — Indicate, S — Specify, C — Consequences).

Example

Health record charts are delivered to the outpatient clinics each morning before the patients arrive for their appointment. The receptionist responsible for assembling each team's charts notes that required and ordered charts are missing. This is occurring with increasing frequency. She documents and reports the problem to the unit director. He decides to take it up with the health records coordinator.

Describe: We have noted over the past three weeks that ordered charts have not been arriving in the outpatient area.

Indicate: This makes patient care very difficult and in some cases impossible since we are functioning without the recorded data and

Specify: I would like a change to occur that would ensure that charts, when ordered, would arrive.

Consequences (*Positive*): That way, we can provide adequate care and stop bothering your staff by requesting charts that didn't come. (*Negative*): If this doesn't occur, it will be necessary to decentralize record keeping so that the charts are in our physical area and thus available to us more quickly. (N.B. Health records is opposed to decentralization of record keeping.)

A DISC Confrontation contains the following:

1. It describes the other person's behavior.
2. It indicates the problems this is causing (but does not refer to your feelings).
3. It specifies what you want the other person to do to improve the situation.
4. It expresses consequences:
    (a) Positive—it points out to the other person the positive result of his complying with your request;
    (b) Negative—If he refuses or seems likely to refuse, it points out the negative results that will occur if he does not comply with your request.

Exercise 38:   Writing a DISC Confrontation

Purpose: To develop skills in writing and making a DISC CONFRONTATION.

Instructions: In pairs, write a DISC CONFRONTATION for the situation described.

Situation

All patient-therapist rooms in the hospital are booked through a central office. You and your patient arrive at the room that has been booked in your name and find it occupied by a health professional student who is studying.

Describe: _____

_____

Indicate: _____

_____

Specify: _____

_____

Consequences:
(Positive): _____

_____

(Negative): _____

_____

Have several pairs role-play their DISC CONFRONTATION for the group.

The type of assertion technique that you use depends on the type of aggressive person that you are dealing with.

With Aggressive People Who:	*Use*
1) Care about you	"I" Confrontation
	DESC Confrontation
2) Don't care about you	DISC Confrontation

D. ACTIVE LISTENING TO CALM AN ANGRY PATIENT

When you assertively confront someone who has been aggressive towards you, he may get defensive and "not hear" what you are saying to him. If the person who is acting aggressively towards you is very upset, you can use the assertive technique of ACTIVE LISTENING to help calm him down. Once he is calm, he will be able to hear your confrontation.

ACTIVE LISTENING is a method of sharing with another person your understanding of what he is trying to say and what he is feeling. Through actively listening to his thoughts and feelings, you are able to reflect back to him in your own words your understanding of what he is saying.

Example

A patient who was brought into the intensive care unit the night before rings his bell. The health professional answers, and the following conversation occurs:

Patient:	Just who do you think you are taking your own sweet time about answering my call? Who's paying you anyway? It's me, Rick Smith, the guy lying here in this bed; so when I ring, you get here fast!
Health professional:	(Thinks: What's gotten into him? I'll try ACTIVE LISTENING.) I hear you saying you're angry because I didn't come quickly enough. (ACTIVE LISTENS)
Patient:	Yeah! Even the guys who can get up and around get faster service than I do.
Health professional:	You're saying everybody else gets things done more quickly than you and that makes you angry. (ACTIVE LISTENS)
Patient:	Yeah! I lie here in this bed and see everybody else doing things and I can't, 'cuz the doctor says I'm sick . . . SICK! I've never been sick a day in my life. I can work harder than anyone.
Health professional:	You're angry about being kept in bed when you don't really feel ill. (ACTIVE LISTENS)
Patient:	Righto! Heart attack! I'm only forty. Forty-year-old men don't have heart attacks. That's for little old men. That's what they die of.
Health professional:	You're frightened of having a problem of this size when you're only forty and you wonder if you're going to die. (ACTIVE LISTENS)
Patient:	(Crying) It's not fair. What am I going to do?

As the above example shows, ACTIVE LISTENING can be used to defuse the anger in an aggressive person's attack on you.

By active listening to the patient, the health professional was able to show the patient she understood his feelings and the situation. This allowed the patient to open up about what was really bothering him—his fear of dying.

When someone is feeling bad and vents his anger on you, ACTIVE LISTENING can be used to get at the real problem. By acting in an understanding manner (showing him you care enough to understand his feelings) an atmosphere of trust develops in which he feels safe to reveal his real feelings. When your patient feels understood he feels good, and this displaces his angry feelings.

Many people are primed for a fight, and they attack you verbally in hope of engaging you in an argument. But it takes two to fight. If you refuse to fight, you eliminate the possibility of your interaction becoming a battleground. If you ACTIVE LISTEN to the aggressive person you may offset the need for a fight by revealing the real source of his anger.

Anger and sadness go together. When someone feels angry, it's often because he feels hurt about something. Aggressive, angry people don't expect understanding. They may feel you don't understand—or worse, don't want to understand, and this is enough to make them feel even angrier. Active Listening can be used to help them express the anger and hurt more constructively. This has a cathartic effect. It helps release pent-up feelings and get rid of them. These emotions can be released constructively or destructively. When you are angry and hit out at someone physically or verbally, you are releasing your anger destructively (aggressively). You have made yourself feel better by hurting someone else. However, if you feel angry, but can express your feelings to someone else, you are releasing your anger constructively. By Active Listening to someone, you show empathy for that person, and he in turn can realize, accept, and express more constructively his feelings.

ACTIVE LISTENING consists of:

1. Restating what the other person is saying (CONTENT REFLECTION)

2. Stating what the other person is feeling (FEELING REFLECTION)

FEELING REFLECTION + CONTENT REFLECTION
= ACTIVE LISTENING

These two components are seen in the last statement of the health professional to the patient.

Health professional: You're frightened, too, (FEELING RE-FLECTION) of having a problem of this size when you're only forty (CONTENT REFLECTION), and you wonder if you're going to die (FEELING REFLECTION).

In some situations, you may want to combine ACTIVE LISTENING with "I" CONFRONTATION. This allows you to assert your rights ("I" CONFRONTATION) while helping the other person express his feelings more constructively (ACTIVE LISTENING). This is a good technique for resolving conflict.

Example

Mr. Jones brings his son to a diagnostic clinic. The nine-year-old boy is obviously small for his chronological age and his upper body seems disproportionately large. A history is obtained and a physical examination done. X-rays and blood work are ordered, and a follow-up appointment made. At the return visit one week later, the following conversation occurs:

Mr. Jones: Well, what's the result?

Health professional: We're still waiting for a result, but . . .

Mr. Jones: You mean you brought me all the way here just to tell me you haven't got the answers?

Health professional: The results we have show no growth glandular dysfunction, and his bone age is appropriate.

Mr. Jones: Damn it! Don't tell me what's right. I wanna know the problem! First you bring me here when you haven't got all the an-swers, then you play around.

Health professional: You're angry because you think you made an unnecessary trip? (ACTIVE LISTENS)

Mr. Jones: Damn right. I know about you guys and how you play around with words.

Health professional: Mr. Jones, when you keep criticizing me I feel frustrated because we're not talking about the real reason you're here—to talk about your son's problems ("I" CONFRON-TATION). This makes me curious, and I wonder if perhaps you're anxious to avoid that. (ACTIVE LISTENING)

Mr. Jones: Of course I wanna know what's wrong.

Health professional: Sometimes it's sad to hear that there aren't any answers or any cures. (ACTIVE LISTENS)

Mr. Jones: I guess . . . I just find it kind of hard to believe my son might not be like other kids.

By alternating "I" CONFRONTATION with ACTIVE LISTENING, the health professional is able to help Mr. Jones express his feelings more assertively. At the same time, the health professional confronts the aggressive approach used by Mr. Jones. ACTIVE LISTENING helps reduce the angry feelings so that the aggressive person can hear what you're really saying. Because you show the other person that you understand how he feels and thinks doesn't mean that you agree with what he has done and said.

E.   COMMON ASSERTION BLOCKS AND HOW TO OVERCOME THEM

It's easy to see that being assertive has payoffs both to the user and the recipient of the message. Recognizing the use of a skill and putting it into practice, however, are two very different things. Often our attempts at being assertive are blocked by ideas that have little foundation in reality but are very relevant to how we feel about ourselves. These assertion blocks are based on certain fears we have: fear of rejection, fear of imperfection in ourselves, and fear of imperfection in others. These blocks may be instrumental in producing nonassertive or aggressive responses when assertive responses would be more productive.

Example

A certain patient is non-compliant with scheduled appointments, yet phones and requests to be seen on short notice for relatively minor problems. The involved health professional always agrees to meet on short notice, and has never discussed the non-compliance with her patient. The health professional would like to confront the patient, but she is afraid he will get angry at her.

We learn early in our careers that a stimulus produces a response. In these situations, we assume that an incident (stimulus) activates a feeling (response). According to psychologist Albert Ellis, our unpleasant feelings are caused not by unpleasant incidents, but by our irrational beliefs about these incidents. In the above example, the incident (stimulus) activates an irrational belief (response). This irrational belief then stimulates a feeling (response). This is illustrated in the diagram below.

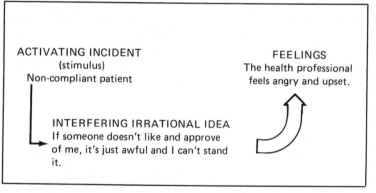

FIGURE 6.1. An Interfering Irrational Idea—Fear of Rejection— Causes Negative Feelings.

Result: The health professional continues to see the patient at a moment's notice, and never discusses the non-attendance.

The irrational components of the health professional's interfering, irrational idea in this example are thoughts like, "It's just awful," and "I can't stand it."

Example

A position has become available in the renal dialysis unit. A health professional has the required qualifications, but decides not to apply although she would like the work. Her reason for not applying is her concern about whether she is the right person for the job.

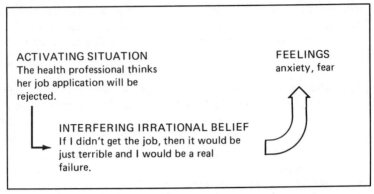

FIGURE 6.2. The Interfering Irrational Belief—Fear of Imperfection.

Result: She does not apply for the position, although she was the best qualified candidate.

The irrational components of her beliefs are statements like: "It would be just terrible," and "I would be a real failure."

Example

A young mother comes to the pediatric well-baby clinic with her two children. Both are being treated for failure to thrive. The mother has required multi-agency input to allow the children to remain with her safely. She proudly announces that she is pregnant. The involved health professional has the following irrational belief about the situation:

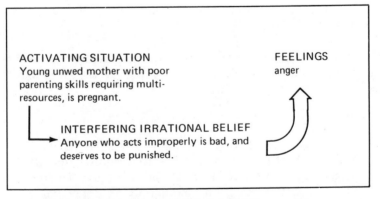

FIGURE 6.3. The Irrational Belief—Intolerance of Imperfection in Others.

Result: The health professional attacks the patient verbally. "What right do you have to have another child? Why don't you have an abortion, or get your tubes tied?"

The irrational components of the health professional's statements were: "is bad" and "deserves to be punished."

Irrational ideas that block assertive action can be dealt with in order to eliminate them, or at least minimize their affecting productivity. First you must identify the activating incident, then identify the associated bad feelings and irrational ideas. Then you must dispute your irrational ideas so that your rational ideas can be identified. These steps are illustrated below using the example of the non-compliant patient.

Example

1. *Identify the Activating Incident:* "Patient is noncompliant and demanding. He missed a scheduled appointment two days ago and called wanting to be seen today for a minor problem. I said yes when I wanted to say no."

2. *Identify Your Bad Feelings:* "I was furious. Who does he think he is—King Tut? I was also afraid that if I said no, he would get angry."

3. *Identify Your Irrational Idea:* "If my patients don't like me and approve of me, then it's just awful. I can't stand it."

4. *Dispute Your Irrational Idea:* "Why is it so awful? Why can't I stand it?"

5. *Identify Your Rational Beliefs About the Situation:*
   (a) "If I were to say no, he probably would get angry."
   (b) "That would be uncomfortable, but not awful."
   (c) "I can withstand it. I've withstood far worse incidents where I've been rejected before."
   (d) "Why should I let my feelings about myself be dependent on whether someone else likes me? I like myself, and that's what's important. If he doesn't like me, I'm still a worthwhile person."
   (e) "This idea (number 3) is irrational—a bunch of nonsense."

(f) "I have a right to say no, and if I do . . ."

(g) who knows? He might even respect me a lot more."

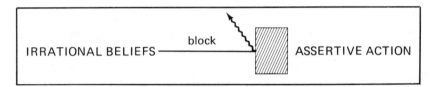

FIGURE 6.4. How Irrational Beliefs Affect Behavior

The three most basic irrational beliefs are:

1. If others don't like me, it's just awful . . . . FEAR OF REJECTION
2. If I'm not perfect, then it's just terrible . . . . FEAR OF IMPERFEC-
   TION (in self)
3. If others make mistakes, then they are . . . . INTOLERANCE OF
   bad, and deserve to be punished by me.   IMPERFECTION IN
   OTHERS

To eliminate your assertion block caused by irrational ideas follow these steps:

1. Identify the activating incident.

2. Identify your bad feelings.

3. Identify your irrational idea.

4. Dispute your irrational idea.

5. Identify your rational beliefs about the situation.

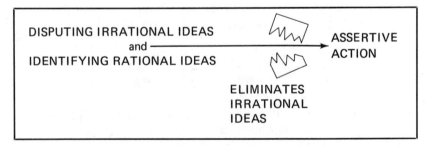

FIGURE 6.5. Effective Action Against Irrational Beliefs.

SUMMARY

Being assertive means expressing your legitimate feelings and rights without hurting others or violating their rights. Assertion is the effective alternative to non-assertive and aggressive behavior. There are seven basic assertion skills: being confrontive, saying no, making requests, expressing opinions, initiating conversations, self-disclosing, and expressing affection. Three assertive confrontation techniques—"I" Confrontation, DESC Confrontation, and DISC Confrontation—are particularly useful for handling conflict situations. By learning how to identify and dispute your irrational ideas you can eliminate your assertion blocks so that you can act in an assertive and effective manner.

7
Developing Skills in Problem-Solving

A. WHAT IS
PROBLEM-SOLVING?

> . . . there are three kinds of things in the world: there are troubles
> which we do not know quite how to handle; then there are
> puzzles with their clear conditions and unique solutions, marvel-
> ously elegant; and then there are problems—and these we invent
> by finding an appropriate puzzle form to impose upon a trouble.

This aphorism has been attributed to the English Platon-
ist, Weldon (Shulman and Elstein 1975), and brings to mind
the different facets of problems. For as much as some problems
can cause discomfort or pain, others challenge, stimulate, and
excite us. Webster's Dictionary says a problem is "anything thrown
forward; a question posed for solution." It is an unsettled situation
that requires the application of knowledge, thought, and skill for
solution. Problem-solving, generally considered the most complex
mental activity known, is an integral part of a health professional's
practice. Without the ability to solve problems effectively, the
health professional's contribution will be limited and he will experience little satisfaction.

Health professionals are involved in different types of problem-
solving. CLINICAL REASONING is one type. In this process, the
health professional transforms a problem (i.e., patient complaints,
signs, and symptoms) into a solution or diagnosis and management plan. This is accomplished by gathering data (such as historical facts, physical examination, and lab investigations), to test out
the various HYPOTHESES (ideas about what is causing the problem) postulated by the health professional. The assessment of clinical reasoning and the educational approach that best teaches and
refines clinical reasoning abilities have received considerable attention in recent years.*

Another type of problem-solving the health professional engages in is within the context of the helping relationship. Here,
the health professional assists the patient in solving his own problem and in making realistic and appropriate plans for change. For
example, a patient has been diagnosed as hypertensive, and medication has been prescribed (the result of CLINICAL REASON-

---

*   H. Barrows and R. Tamblyn, undated monograph no. 1; E. Berner, T.
Bligh, and R. Guerin, 1977; J. Bjorn and H. Cross, 1970; J. Feightner, H.
Barrows, and V. Neufeld, 1977; A. Feinstein, 1974; J. Hurst and H.
Walker, 1972; J. Marshall, 1977; C. McGuire, 1976; L. Shulman and A.
Elstein, 1975; P. Ways, G. Loftus, and J. Jones, 1973; H. Simon and A.
Newell, 1970).

ING). But the patient keeps forgetting to take the medication. In this situation, the health professional would help the patient explore various alternatives and decide on the plan that would most likely solve the problem (i.e., help the patient remember the medication).

There are many situations where a health professional is a member or leader of a group that is trying to solve a problem. This may be a team planning management for a patient or a group of health professionals planning for clinic expansion. Problem-solving in groups is somewhat different from assisting one individual with this process, and the health professional will be better able to facilitate the process if he has an understanding of groups and group dynamics.

This chapter addresses the last two types of problem solving: problem-solving with a patient or another health professional and problem-solving in groups.

B. STEPS IN PROBLEM-SOLVING

For problem-solving to be successful and the desired outcome reached, there must be a systematic approach used. This approach includes the following steps:

1. Sense a problem
2. Define the problem
3. Identify alternative solutions
4. Consider the consequences of the different solutions
5. Choose a solution
6. Carry out the plan
7. Evaluate the outcome

1. Sense a Problem

When a problem exists, those involved initially experience a vague sense of discomfort or uneasiness. Something is "just not right." Some cue, such as a change in behavior or a behavior that is incongruent with a statement, triggers this feeling. Often heard is the comment, "I knew something was wrong the minute I entered the room." In this case, the cue may have been the absence of talking in a group that was usually quite vocal. Once aware of this feeling, a person becomes more sensitive to other incoming messages, which could confirm or refute that initial sense of discomfort. A data gathering process occurs that might include further observation, direct questioning, or recall of past knowledge or past experience. To continue with the previous example, the person who entered the room might have then observed angry looks on the faces and recalled that this group had frequently been unable to resolve conflicts. Yes, there is a problem. Having confirmed that a problem exists, the next step is to define the problem.

2. Define the Problem

Once it has been established that a problem does exist, data collection continues because several questions must be answered:

> Where is the problem?
> What is the problem?
> Why does the problem exist?

Identifying *where* the problem is means discovering whether it rests within an individual (e.g., poor compliance with a therapy plan), between individuals (e.g., role conflict between two different health professionals), within a group (e.g., poor commitment to the group), or within a system (e.g., overly stringent rules). *What* the problem is should then be decided. This requires careful consideration because it is often easy to confuse the result of the problem (the obvious manifestation) with the real problem. Table 7.1 illustrates this difference.

TABLE 7.1

WHERE the problem is	MANIFESTATION of the problem	WHAT the problem is
Individual	Obese patient	Poor compliance with diet
Between individuals	Two health professionals always arguing	Role conflict
Group	Poor group attendance	Lack of commitment to group
System	Disgruntled and angry staff	Overly stringent rules

The next question to ask is, "*Why* does the problem exist?" Problems usually exist because of unmet needs. The more accurate the health professional is in identifying the unmet need, the more likely reasonable solutions will be generated. For example, the health professional interviewed 17-year-old Colleen about her problem—failure to comply with a prescribed low calorie diet. The health professional discovered that Colleen felt isolated from her peers and in order to feel more a part of the group, joined them daily at the local fast food place. The unmet need was a sense of belonging. By eating wih the group, Colleen met this need. Table 7.2 illustrates this with the other examples.

TABLE 7.2

WHERE the problem is	MANIFESTA- TION of the problem	WHAT the problem is	Unmet need
Individual	Obese patient	Poor compliance with diet	Sense of belonging
Between individuals	Two health professionals always arguing	Role conflict	To be in control
Group	Poor group attendance	Lack of commitment to group	Sense of purpose
System	Disgruntled and angry staff	Overly stringent rules	Opportunities for creativity

When looking for the "*why*," the health professional should consider a wide range of possibilities. Including the patient in this process is important since it is necessary for the health professional and the patient to agree on why the problem exists. A clear statement of the problem completes this step.

3.   Identify Alternative Solutions

After defining the problem, alternative solutions should be generated. Avoid being "solution-minded" and feeling satisfied after proposing one solution. Push on to another solution and for yet another. Use different ideas for each solution. Using this approach, one is more likely to be creative. Recalling what was tried before and what was good about that plan may also prove helpful. For example, solutions, for Colleen's problem could be:

1.   not meeting the group at the fast food place;
2.   going, but only drinking a low calorie drink;
3.   going and eating, but increasing the amount of exercise;
4.   altering the diet to allow for some "fast food" on certain days;
5.   planning a "reward" for every day she goes but refrains from eating or drinking;
6.   leaving her money at home so she is unable to make a food purchase;
7.   educating her about the value of good nutrition;
8.   joining another group activity that does not include eating;
9.   inviting a friend or group of friends home.

4.   Evaluate the Alternatives

The consequences of each proposed solution should be explored. "What will happen if this is done?" is the question to ask. Frequently, this will point to one or two better choices. For example: if Colleen decided not to meet her friends at the fast food place she might avoid the temptation to eat. However, she might also miss out on valuable social interaction that meets her belonging need.

5.   Choose a Solution

Those involved in the problem then decide on a solution and who will be responsible for carrying out what part of the plan. For example, Colleen decided that the best plan for her was to eat selectively at the fast food place and increase her exercising accordingly. The health professional's tasks were to list the caloric content of each food and list exercises and the number of calories used with each one. The health professional would call Colleen in one week to answer any questions and offer encouragement. Colleen's tasks were to choose the food with fewer calories and to do the exercises. She would return to the clinic in two weeks to be weighed and to discuss her progress.

6.   Carry Out the Plan

Colleen continued to attend the fast food place, but chose foods more nutritionally suitable for her dietary plan. She chose a green salad or yogurt rather than a hamburger and french fries. Instead of busing the two miles to school, she began walking. She joined a swimming class in the evenings. She compiled her list of foods for the health professional and was diligent about carrying out her exercises. Colleen and the health professional met after two weeks to review Colleen's progress. He determined the caloric content of the foods Colleen had listed and suggested some additional exercises she could try out. She was weighed.

7.   Evaluate the Outcome

Did the chosen plan of action solve the problem? Was it a reasonable and workable choice? What were the good parts about the plan? Are any mid-course corrections needed? How might this solution be applied to other problems?

   After four weeks Colleen had lost five pounds and was enthusiastic about the support her friends were giving her. They were following her lead in changing their own diets and were eating less starchy foods. Several had remarked on her improved respiratory status. Since beginning the diet and exercise, Colleen was able to climb the three flights of stairs at school without puffing—for her a feat indeed!

   These seven steps constitute the problem-solving process.

Exercise 39:   Identifying Steps in Problem-Solving

Purpose: To identify the steps in problem-solving.

Instructions: 1.   Read the following situation.

   Sam was a health professional student who was assigned to the post-partum unit to care for a woman and her newborn baby. His instructor observed that he was tense and extremely awkward in his handling of the baby. The instructor considered the possible reasons for his behavior: no previous experience with newborns, no previous experience on a postpartum unit, past bad experience, lack of knowledge about newborn behavior, general clumsiness, presence of instructor, concern about his male image, or outside factor causing increased stress. The instructor went on a coffee break with the student.

Instructor:	How is the morning going?
Student:	So-so.
Instructor:	In what way, so-so?
Student:	Well, I'm nervous about handling newborns.
Instructor:	What about handling them makes you uneasy?
Student:	The mother watching me. On my last day in pediatrics, a mother walked in while I was trying to pull a shirt over her baby's head. She really got upset and made a scene because I wasn't "doing it right."
Instructor:	Are you afraid this mother will get upset and embarrass you, too?
Student:	Yes.

They discussed different ways of handling the student's concern. Some of them were: assist Sam with his unresolved feelings about the previous experience, remove the newborn to the nursery when care was being provided, have the instructor explore the mother's feelings about the care being provided for her new baby, have Sam spend more time getting to know the mother. After discussing the pro's and con's of the various possibilities, Sam decided on the last alternative. He also wanted to discuss his previous experience with his instructor at a later time. At the end of the clinical rotation, Sam and his instructor met for evaluation. Sam felt the problem had been resolved; the instructor's recent observations concurred with his statement. They discussed which parts of their plan had been most helpful to him.

> 2. Put a * where the problem was sensed. What type(s) of data gathering occurred?

_____

_____

> 3. Define the problem.

_____

_____

> 4. Identify the remaining steps of problem-solving.

_____

_____

C.   FACTORS THAT INFLUENCE PROBLEM-SOLVING

There are many factors influencing a health professional's problem-solving. Some of these are educational background, knowledge base, and degree of understanding of human behavior. For example, many children are afraid to go to the dentist. A dentist with no education in child development and behavior will solve the problem of the frightened child one way. He may see sedation as the answer. The dentist who has had courses in childhood development may solve the problem by preparing the child for the experience. He may mail an information sheet to the parents explaining the importance of telling the child what to expect. Included may be a comic book about going to the dentist. Toys and storybooks might be placed in the waiting room. A parent would be allowed to stay with the child while the dentist worked. In this example, one can see that education influences the health professional's ability to generate alternative solutions.

How a health professional perceives his role in relation to patients will determine aspects of problem-solving. For example, Dr. Taylor sees her role primarily as a skilled surgeon. She defines patient problems within that context: bowel obstruction, cancer of the stomach, peritoneal abscess. Compare this to Dr. McCarthy, another surgeon. He sees his role as operating on patients and helping them adjust to any lifestyle changes that may need to be made. His definition of a patient problem would be broader. It would include physical, psychological, and emotional components.

How a health professional perceives his role in relation to colleagues also influences the problem-solving process. The nurse who perceives other professionals as being more knowledgeable and important, may spend much time gathering data from them when attempting to solve a nursing problem. It may be difficult for her to "pick a solution" independently without first consulting others for their opinion. Her perception of her role as being in some way "less" than her colleagues will prevent efficient problem-solving.

Past experience with a similar problem, successful or unsuccessful, is another factor. The health professional who views an unsuccessful problem-solving experience as a method failure and not a personal failure, will be able to approach similar problems more constructively in the future. Personal attitudes and values,

interest in the problem, commitment to finding a solution, tolerance for human differences, and willingness to take risks also
influence the problem-solving process.

Exercise 40:   Factors Influencing Problem Identification

Purpose: To identify factors that influence problem identification.

Instructions: 1.   Read the following situation.

Katrina, a 19-year-old single woman, brought her 2-year-old son,
David, to a well-child clinic for a routine check-up. When asked by
the health professional if she had any concerns, she replied, "He
won't eat." Since his last check-up, he had not been ill, but he
had been to the emergency room twice for stitches and once for
head trauma (without loss of consciousness). His diet was normal
for his age. The rest of the history was unremarkable. Katrina was
completing high school during the day and had a babysitter for
David. The physical and developmental exam showed an active,
curious 2-year-old with no abnormalities.

(a) Identify the patient problems as you see
them.

_____

_____

_____

_____

_____

(b) Which problem do you feel needs attention
first?

_____

(c) Which problem is of least concern?

_____

2.   Share your responses in pairs, noting similarities and differences in your problem lists. Identify reasons for the differences.
Do they reflect different health professional
roles?
Do they reflect different past experiences?

Do they reflect areas of personal interest and/or
expertise?
Do they reflect different values?

A major factor in problem-solving with a patient or within a
group is the health professional's ability to communicate.
PROBLEM-SOLVING INTERPERSONAL SKILLS are necessary
for efficient and successful problem-solving. For example, OB-
SERVATION SKILLS make the health professional more sensitive
to incongruent messages; this facilitates early problem identification.

Example

Mrs. Barnes has brought 3-month old Jon to the clinic
for a minor cold. She tells the health professional that
she is not worried but thought it would be a good idea
to have him checked anyway. She has a frown on her
face and seems close to tears. She is unable to look at
the health professional directly.

Health professional: You tell me you are not worried, but you
seem pretty upset today. (OBSERVA-
TION). Is there something else you'd like
to tell me or ask me?

Mrs. Barnes: I try so hard to do everything right, but he
keeps getting sick. What am I doing wrong?

In this situation the health professional was able to help Mrs.
Barnes express her real concern by OBSERVING the discrepancies between her words and her facial expression. OBSERVATION
SKILLS also provide information about how the problem-solving
process is affecting an individual or group.

Example

Mrs. Porter brought 4-year-old Linda to the clinic for a
regular check-up. Linda sat quietly while the health
professional took her history until the question of bed-
wetting was raised. It seems that this had been an ongoing problem. The health professional began to pursue
possible approaches with the mother. At this time,
Linda got up and started opening and closing the cup-
board and interrupting her mother with questions. The

health professional OBSERVED the behavior and commented that Linda seemed very uncomfortable. The health professional then reassured the child and included her more directly in the problem solving.

CLARIFICATION SKILLS (seeking a more detailed explanation) assist with defining the problem, identifying alternative solutions, and considering the consequences of the solutions. Some useful questions to ask might be: "What do you mean by that?" "How did you arrive at that conclusion?" "What do you think will happen if the patient tries that solution?" EXPRESSING AN OPINION is a useful skill when the consequences of the different alternatives are being discussed. After a solution has been chosen, MAKING A REQUEST is a skill that helps with delegating the tasks. The last step, EVALUATING THE OUTCOME, utilizes all of these interpersonal skills. ACTIVE LISTENING is perhaps the single most valuable interpersonal skill in problem-solving. It can be used effectively in each of the seven steps of the process.

Exercise 41:   Problem-Solving Interpersonal Skills

Purpose: To practice using INTERPERSONAL SKILLS for problem solving.

Instructions: This exercise requires three people—one to be a health professional, one to be a patient with a problem, and one to be an observer.

1(a)   The "patient" decides on a simple problem to take to the health professional. Perhaps he portrays a parent with a child having behavior problems. Perhaps he portrays a patient who keeps forgetting to take his medication.

(b)   The health professional helps the patient solve the problem.

(c)   The observer notes the INTERPERSONAL SKILLS used throughout the problem solving and places a check in the appropriate space each time one of the INTERPERSONAL SKILLS is used.

2.   At the end of the problem-solving process, the observer should show the health professional and patient how many INTERPERSONAL SKILLS were used.

Interpersonal Skill	Place a Check (✓) When Used
1. ACTIVE LISTENING	_____
2. CLARIFICATION	_____
3. EXPRESSING AN OPINION	_____
4. MAKING A REQUEST	_____
5. OBSERVATION	_____
6. OTHER (SPECIFY)	_____
_____	

Questions for Discussion

- How did the "patient" feel during the interview? Can this be related to the use (or non-use) of interpersonal skills?

- Did the "patient" feel the problem was resolved? If not, why?

- Discuss any specific recommendations you have for the "health professional."

Exercise 42:   Solving Problems Together

Purposes: To identify a problem and decide on a management plan with another health professional.
To identify the PROBLEM-SOLVING INTER-PERSONAL SKILLS that facilitated the task.

Instructions: 1.   Read the following situation.

Mr. O'Hara was seen in the family practice unit three weeks ago for a regular check-up. At the time it was noted that he had a chronic cough. A skin test for tuberculosis was applied. When the health professional called him for the result, the description Mr. O'Hara gave made it sound like there had been a significant skin reaction. He was scheduled to return to the unit that day, but did not. Several subsequent appointments were not kept as well.

(a) With another health professional, identify the problem.

(b) Together, decide what steps should be taken to resolve the problem, and who in the situation should be responsible for the various tasks.

_____

_____

_____

_____

(c) Identify the PROBLEM-SOLVING INTERPERSONAL SKILLS that facilitated how you and your partner completed the task.

_____

_____

_____

_____

D.   COMMON BLOCKS TO PROBLEM-SOLVING

One of the most common blocks to problem-solving is failure to make use of the information we already have. In *Organizational Psychology: A Book of Readings* by Kolb, Rubin, and McIntyre, readers are reminded of an old story that illustrates this point. A truck became stuck in an underpass. A variety of solutions, all including major alterations of the truck or underpass, were offered by onlookers. Then, a small boy suggested letting the air out of the tires. The others had focussed only on the top of the truck and did not make use of the other readily available information.

Premature closure is another common block. This occurs when a solution is decided on before all alternative solutions have been identified and evaluated. Past failures with similar problems may limit one's ability to see what is new in the current situation. If the problem does not make sense, the natural tendency is to focus on one of the elements that does make sense. If it is the wrong element, the problem will not be solved.

Lastly, poor INTERPERSONAL SKILLS hamper problem-solving when it is done with another individual or in a group.

Exercise 43:   Premature Closure

Purpose: To demonstrate how choosing a solution before *all* alternative solutions have been considered limits your creativity or ability to see alternative solutions in case the first one fails.

Instructions: 1.   Read the following situation.

Barclay was 3-years-old and very obese. He lived with his mother, teenage brother, and grandparents. His obesity was due to the fact that people in his environment were feeding him all the time.

Solution to the problem: A home visit by the nutritionist to discuss nutritional needs of a 3-year-old and to help develop a diet.

   (a) The above solution failed to solve the problem. Identify alternative solutions.

_____

_____

_____

   (b) As a group or individually, consider the following question: As you searched for alternative solutions, did you find yourself thinking about the previous solution and seeing all subsequent solutions within that same context (e.g., educating the family)?

   2(a) Divide the group into two subgroups. Give each subgroup a brief description of a new health care problem. Give only one group a solution to the problem.

   (b) Allow 15 minutes for each group to list alternative solutions to the problem.

   (c) Compare the two lists and discuss.

   Were there differences in the scope of solutions presented? Did a "mind set" prevent the group that was initially given a solution from being creative in proposing alternative solutions?

E.   PROBLEM-SOLVING
IN GROUPS

A health professional is frequently a member of a group that is involved in problem-solving. Using the seven problem-solving steps is still necessary if good solutions are to be found. All of the previously mentioned factors that influence problem-solving (e.g., perception of role, past experience, values) are applicable to group problem solving since a group is a collection of individuals. The added factor is the system of interaction among the various group members. This makes the group quantitatively and qualitatively different from the individual members. The group membership, norms, goals, authority structure, leadership, and communication patterns must be considered. All these elements affect group problem-solving. For example, if the group membership consists of all nurses, role conflict (between different types of health professionals) will not exist in the group. Problem-solving in a group whose norms are promptness and "no socializing" will be different from that in a group whose norms are more laissez-faire in the areas of punctuality and socializing. The first may be more efficient in getting to the task at hand. Members of the second group may feel more relaxed about expressing their opinions.

Exercise 44:   Group Observation

Purpose: To identify how group membership, norms, and goals affect the problem-solving of the group.

Instructions: Think about a group you are in. Make the following observations.

1(a) What is the group membership?

_____

(b) How does the membership affect the group's ability to problem solve?

_____

_____

2(a) What group norms facilitate the problem-solving?

_____

_____

(b) Are there any norms which make problem-solving more difficult?

_____

_____

3(a) What are the group's goals?

_____

_____

(b) How do these goals affect problem-solving?

_____

_____

4. Share your responses in pairs.

You may find that in one group the goals are not clearly defined and that the motivation for problem-solving is low.

You may find that some of the norms are very supportive of the problem-solving process, while other norms (e.g., long discussions on every point) make problem-solving more difficult.

Compare and contrast the groups you and your partner observed.

Certain factors facilitate problem-solving in a group. A climate that is accepting and non-judgmental permits group members to express opinions, concerns, and desires. A group that has a strong common purpose is usually more motivated to solve a problem.

For example, a health care team that has a common purpose of providing excellent patient care will be motivated to resolve patient problems. A group whose members are divided in purpose between patient care and research may have less motivation to resolve patient problems. When the individual members feel responsible for reaching a solution and for using everyone's ideas, problem-solving is facilitated.

There are certain roles within the group that facilitate problem-solving. One role is that of INITIATOR. The INITIATOR is active in proposing tasks or goals and in identifying problems. He begins the problem-solving process. Another role is the INFOR-MATION SEEKER. This group member asks others for facts and opinions relevant to the problem and requests clarification of statements. This results in the pooling of ideas, opinions, and knowledge from all the members. Confusion is prevented or cleared up. The complementary role is INFORMATION GIVER; this is alternately taken by various contributing members. Another role, that of SUMMARIZER, is important for pulling related ideas together. He reminds the group of where they are in the problem-solving process by making statements like, "The problem has been defined as . . . ." or "So far, we have considered the pro's and con's of two of the solutions, and they are . . . ." He is responsible for presenting to the group a decision or proposed solution, thereby pushing the group to take the first step toward reaching a consensus. The CONSENSUS TESTER then questions the group members about the reality of the proposed solution and its prac-ticality. He checks with the different group members to see how much agreement exists. If there is agreement among the members, consensus has been reached and the tasks related to the decision are then delegated. If there is no consensus, the group returns to an earlier stage in the problem-solving process and the other facili-tative roles again become important.

One group member may have more than one role. The same person may function as an INITIATOR and later as a CONSEN-SUS TESTER, or as INFORMATION SEEKER and SUMMA-RIZER. These roles are not assigned, but rather tend to evolve as the group attempts to problem-solve. A well functioning group is characterized by all of these roles being assumed by its members.

Exercise 45:   Facilitating Group Development

Purpose: To identify factors in a group that facilitate problem-solving.

To identify which members took facilitative roles.

Instructions: This exercise requires a group of 8 people, 2 of whom are observers, and a facilitator.

1.   Read the following situation.

Mary is an R.N. with a B.S. degree and is the charge nurse on a surgical unit during the night shift. Every morning Celia, a nursing assistant, begins waking the patients at 5:00 a.m. to weigh them and take their temperatures. She usually completes this by 6:00 a.m. The shift ends at 8:00 a.m. Mary has repeatedly asked Celia to wait until 7:00 a.m. to do this task to allow patients more time to sleep. But Celia persists in beginning at 5:00 a.m.

(a) The group is given 20 minutes to solve the problem.

(b) While the group is problem solving, the first observer writes down what factors are facilitating the process.

_____

_____

_____

_____

_____

_____

(c) The second observer notes who takes which role by placing a check mark in the appropriate space each time a group member displays a particular role.

Names of Group Members

Role						
1. Initiator						
2. Information Seeker						
3. Information Giver						
4. Summarizer						
5. Consensus Taker						

2.   At the end of the 20 minutes, the group should discuss the following questions.

Questions for Discussion

- How does the group feel they did?
- Was the problem solved?
- What factors facilitated getting the task done?
- Who within the group took a facilitative role? Identify the nature of the role.

3. The observers share their observations with the group, and the group decides whether there is agreement between the group's perception of what transpired and the observers' perception. Discuss any discrepancies.

F. BLOCKS TO PROBLEM-SOLVING IN GROUPS

Many groups lack knowledge of or appreciation for the problem-solving process. One result may be a poorly defined problem. It may not be stated in concrete terms or take into account the *where, what,* and *why.* It is very difficult to solve a problem that has not been defined. Another result is that these groups tend to develop rapid and premature solutions. Few alternative solutions are explored. Discussion of the consequences of the proposed solutions may be haphazard. Incomplete use of all the resources in the group may be another factor that limits the number and scope of alternative solutions that are generated.

Failure to reach a consensus about the solution is another block to problem-solving. Unless all group members agree to at least try the solution, commitment to the various tasks that need to be done will be low. Those who strongly disagree with the solution may subtly undermine the efforts of the rest of the group.

Poor problem-solving methods do limit a group's success in getting a task done. Just as often, though, the problems that prove most disruptive and cause the greatest loss of time and energy are the result of poor interpersonal relationships. Interpersonal skills—HELPING SKILLS, BEHAVIOR CHANGE SKILLS, PROBLEM-SOLVING INTERPERSONAL SKILLS, ASSERTION SKILLS—facilitate task accomplishment. The health professional who has good INTERPERSONAL SKILLS and a solid understanding of the steps in problem-solving will be better able to manage the situations that confront him throughout his career.

SUMMARY

Health professionals are constantly faced with problems to be solved. In order to do this efficiently and effectively, it is important to establish and follow a pattern for problem-solving that produces results. The key steps in problem-solving are:

1. Sense a problem
2. Define the problem
3. Identify alternative solutions
4. Consider the consequences of the different solutions
5. Choose a solution
6. Carry out the plan
7. Evaluate the outcome

By being aware of those factors that either block or facilitate problem-solving, the health professional is able to promote more effective care of his patients.

8

Developing Skills in Understanding Group, Team, and Organizational Behavior

Health care involves an interaction between at least two individuals—a client-patient, or health care seeker, and a health care professional or provider. For efficient and effective health care to be provided for any individual or group of people, a multitude of persons are necessary. These persons may be government employees regulating the standards within which health care is provided; they may be lab technicians participating in the manufacture of medication for disease entities; or they may be health professionals providing primary care at the bedside or in the community. An organization is required for the provision of effective health care. This health care organization has similarities with all other organizations.

An organization consists of subunits that are formally differentiated along various lines (Blau and Schoenherr 1971). Organizing is determining, assembling, and arranging the resources by function and in relation to the whole to meet the planned objective (Appley, 1952). Successful organizations have certain characteristics. They have clearly defined responsibilities or GOALS. They have strong resourceful LEADERSHIP. They have a carefully selected, appropriately trained, and strategically placed workforce (ROLES). They have standardized procedures and documentation methods. They have an adequate financial base. They have co-operation between group members which produces a productive CLIMATE and effective COMMUNICATION.

Throughout this chapter, the aforementioned concepts will be examined using a patient care model.

Example

Mrs. Jones and her 5-year-old daughter, Josephine, have been flown to a pediatric specialty hospital several hundred miles from their small hometown. Josephine's problems were extensive—a cardiac defect, juvenile rheumatoid arthritis, a hearing defect, and growth retardation. The trip had been precipitated by a severe electrolyte imbalance.

When Josie's home community of three hundred people learned that she would be hospitalized for an additional several months, they mobilized themselves to aid the Jones family. This fishing village, a group by virtue of the fact that all members of the town knew or were related to Josie, became organized. The GOAL was to provide financial assistance to allow Mrs. Jones to accompany Josie to the distant hospital and remain with her throughout the additional hospitalization. The chosen LEADER was the village priest, a man well-respected in the community. Meetings were held to develop fund-raising schemes. The fishermen decided to offer two days' fishing income to the family. The merchants gave the profits of one day's sales. The home-makers held a bake sale with all proceeds going to the Josie fund. In this CLIMATE of caring and sharing the community gathered sufficient monies to support the Jones' family through a three-month hospitalization. The goal having been achieved, the organization disbanded. The group remained actively interested in Josie's progress.

A. GOALS

A GOAL is that state or direction towards which an individual or group strives. Goals usually emerge in response to unmet needs. The purpose of the goal is to alleviate the need. Thus, the goal is the endpoint, but a process must occur for the goal to be reached. This process is called PROBLEM-SOLVING. When the problem is solved, the goal has been reached.

Goals have many functions. First, they establish a standard or common objective towards which the group strives. Therefore, the group's effort becomes more directed, co-ordinated, and rational.

Example

The goal of the health care team involved in caring for Josephine was to investigate, diagnose, and treat Josie's problems in the best manner possible while allowing for her maximum potential and dignity.

The goal of Josephine's mother was to keep her daughter alive and expose her to the least amount of trauma possible.

Josephine's goal was to avoid pain and keep Mommy as close as possible. The head nurse's goal was to encourage an interdisciplinary approach to attainment of the team goal.

Second, the goal becomes a source of identification for the individual and the group and may be a motivator. When individuals can relate their own personal objectives or goals to that of the group goal, they will be more motivated to reach the group goal. However, if the individual's goals are in opposition to the goals of the group or organization, conflict is produced and must be resolved.

Example

The hospital had always used a strong authoritarian leadership which allowed little room for formal sharing amongst disciplines. If that pattern were used for attainment of the team goal, then the head nurse's goal of interdisciplinary communication would not be achieved. Since the head nurse was in a position to influence a climate to either facilitate or sabotage the efforts to reach the goal, discrepancies between the head nurse's goal and the goal of the hospital administration would have to be resolved.

GOAL INTEGRATION occurs when members of a team or organization are able to meet both personal goals and institutional objectives through the activities assigned within the institution. This can occur in several ways. Either the individual can be socialized to want to meet the goals of the institution or the organizational procedures can be modified to accommodate the individual so that he can meet his goals.

Example

Since attainment of the long-term goals was going to incur some pain for Josie, it was necessary that there be alteration of either the team goals or her mother's goal with regard to pain for Josie. In this situation, both goals were altered slightly. The team incorporated a program of explanations and play therapy into their treatment approach. This minimized Josie's fear and provided her with an outlet for fear and anxiety. Mrs. Jones altered her goal to incorporate an understanding of the need for certain painful procedures, and she made a decision to support Josie while allowing the treatments to occur.

B. ROLES

Certain behaviors are expected from a person having a particular position or status in a group or organization. Position means the place occupied within the group. Status means the rank or importance of the place occupied. The sum total of these behaviors is called the role. The individual occupying the role must be content with the role and its social norms and these behaviors must be compatible with the individual's personal needs. Otherwise, role conflict occurs. The role of any one individual in a group is determined in part by personal expectations and in part by group expectations. Unclear or ambiguous role expectations of other group members can result in disharmony and conflict. ROLE AMBIGUITY can occur if other team members' expectations of an individual are not made clear to that individual.

Example

The ward dietician became involved in individual situations only when referrals were made to her. These referrals came infrequently and, in the dietician's opinion, often inappropriately. She was aware of Josie's presence on the ward and of her multitude of problems, including failure to thrive. She was also aware that Josie would require high protein reserves to prepare her for the pending surgery. When no referral was made, she began to alter the child's diet sheets to provide for a higher protein menu. This was done without the knowledge of the mother or the team caring for Josie. Mrs. Jones' frustrated comment that the menu received was not what was ordered persuaded the staff to examine the situation. They recognized that a dietary consultation was appropriate but, by not formally making a referral, the dietician was placed in an ambiguous position as was the mother, child, and staff.

ROLE AMBIGUITY occurs if a team member is not sure what he should be doing, is not sure what other members of the team think he should be doing, and is not sure what other team members should be doing.

ROLE CONFLICT occurs when other team members make demands of you that are not harmonious with your expectations of yourself and when other team members make demands that are not harmonious with each other.

Example

Mrs. Jones had studied child development and had worked for a period of time in a child recreation program. She enjoyed the work, and, since Josie's hospitalization, had often assisted the child life staff in the playroom. Since the child life program was very short staffed, Mrs. Jones' help was greatly appreciated. In fact, staff began to rely on it. This caused conflict for Mrs. Jones when she realized that her role as a mother and a support for Josie was being hindered by her volunteer work.

ROLE OVERLOAD would have resulted if Mrs. Jones had felt it was necessary to do both jobs equally well. When role conflict, role ambiguity, or role overload occur there may be ROLE RENEGOTIATION. This is a "give and take" to facilitate more co-operative and efficient team functioning.

It may be necessary to role negotiate many times during a team's existence. In order to do so, there must first be an assessment of role expectations. This involves each member sharing his expectations. At this point, role conflicts and role ambiguity may be revealed, and then alternative solutions can be negotiated. This requires a problem-solving session to arrive at the best and most workable solutions. At this point, it is often advantageous to implement a ROLE CONTRACT (i.e., a contract amongst the team members specifying role expectations agreed to by all parties). An evaluation of the negotiated contract should occur at an agreed upon time. The criteria examined may include: quality and quantity of work being produced, observable aspects of the team members' behavior, and feelings individuals have about themselves and other members of the health care team.

In summary, role negotiation requires that certain steps take place:

1. ASSESSMENT: Identifying that a problem exists and assessing its parameters. This includes identifying role conflicts, role ambiguity, and role overload.

2. ANALYSIS: Alternative solutions to the problem must be generated.

3. CHOICE: After negotiation, the best alternative is chosen.

4. ACTION: The solution is implemented.

5. EVALUATION: The outcome is assessed.

Role negotiation is essentially a problem-solving process. It is described in greater detail elsewhere in the text.

Exercise 46: Roles and Tasks

Purpose: To examine role definition, role negotiation, and role overlap.

Instructions: 1. Select four persons to form a small group. The remainder of the group functions as observers.

2. The small group is to role-play the situation described below. Each person in the group is to role-play one of the health professional roles.

3. On completion of ten minutes of role-playing, a chairperson is to lead the group in examining topics related to the roles played.

Situation

Four individuals have been hired by a hospital to provide secondary paediatric assessment. Although they have never met before, the institution expects them to function in an interdisciplinary manner using a team approach. The four professionals are: paediatrician, paediatric nurse-practitioner, social worker, and child life-worker. This is their first meeting, and their goal is to negotiate roles.

Questions for Discussion

- As a group, how did you role negotiate the selection of chairman? What roles did group members play, and how was this determined?

- Was any attempt made to define the roles of each health professional?

- Did any role overlapping occur? Did this create conflict? How was this handled?

C. AUTHORITY

AUTHORITY refers to the acceptance of the directives of others because they are thought to be legitimate. Authority can also be defined as the right to take actions (Hicks 1972). Stieglitz (1972) refers to organizational principles relating to authority. Specifically:

1. There should be clear lines of authority running from the top to the bottom of the organization and accountability from bottom to top.

2.   The responsibility and authority of each position should be clearly defined in writing.

3.   Accountability should always be coupled with corresponding authority.

4.   Authority to take or initiate action should be delegated as close to the scene of action as possible.

5.   The number of levels of authority should be kept to a minimum.

Authority can be: (1) formal, official, or positional; or (2) functional or personal.

Formal authority is vested in the position held by the individual. It is a mechanism enabling the leader to direct the work of others. Formal authority involves both the AUTHORITY OF LEGITIMACY and the AUTHORITY OF THE POSITION. Authority of legitimacy accounts for subordinates deferring to authority because it is authority, while authority of the position derives from the acknowledged status inherent in the official role or position.

Formal, positional, or official authority is constant. While incumbent directors of health care may come and go, the position with its inherent authority remains. Although positional authority implies the power to direct and make decisions for subordinates, the job to be done must be accomplished by these same subordinates. They potentially can undermine the efforts of the authority figure by refusing (overtly or covertly) to support his decision. Therefore, the job may not be accomplished.

Functional or personal authority derives from the personal qualities of the individual leader. In health care settings, the most valued personal qualities are professional competence, experience, technical experience, knowledge of managerial functions and human relations, and an understanding and use of POWER. Although an individual may have no formal positional authority, his functional personal authority may allow him to wield a great deal of influence.

Power, which is important for functional or personal authority, can be defined as the ability and willingness to affect the behavior of others (Claus and Bailey, 1977).

Since anyone participating in a group, team, or organization will be subject to both authority and power, it is advantageous to recognize the differences between formal and functional authority. The real lines of power and authority in organizations are often not the formal ones.

Exercise 47:   Organizational Authority

Purpose: To examine your place in your organization's authority structure.

Instructions: 1.   On your own, complete the Organizational Authority Inventory. Place a check (✓) in the space which best describes your response to the following questions.

ORGANIZATIONAL AUTHORITY INVENTORY

	A Great Deal	A Moderate Amount	A Small Amount
1. How much authority do you have in your organization?			
2. How much have you participated in setting goals and policies in your organization			
3. Do you know the duties that are part of your job role?			
4. Do you observe the rules of your organization?			
5. Do you have influence with your employer?			
6. Is your influence accepted by your superior?			

2.   How satisfied are you in your organization? Check (✓) the appropriate spot on. the line below.

very
satisfied _____ very
unsatisfied

3.   In pairs, share your responses.

Questions for Discussion

• What is the relationship between the amount of authority you have in your organization and your feelings of satisfaction?

- What would you have to change to obtain more authority?
- Are you aware of persons who have authority in your organization, not by virtue of their formal job role, but by virture of the personal influence they have on other people?

D. LEADERSHIP

Leadership is important for enabling team members to be their most effective. The following types of leadership are familiar to health professionals:

AUTHORITARIAN
LAISSEZ-FAIRE
DEMOCRATIC

1. Authoritarian Leadership

An AUTHORITARIAN leadership style involves the leader taking responsibility for all decision making. He thereafter delegates tasks to group members and may be instrumental in assigning roles to people. The AUTHORITARIAN leader is not required to take the opinions of other team members into consideration, and he expects complete obedience to the decisions he makes. This style is familiar to most health professionals since it is the traditional method of providing health care. Usually, a physician is the AUTHORITARIAN leader who diagnoses the illness and prescribes the treatment for the patient to accept and other health professionals to provide. One disadvantage of AUTHORITARIAN leadership is that it may lead to arbitrary decisions that result in poorer health for the patient.

Example

Dr. Brown had grown up in the traditional setting where the physician's word was final. In the situation with Josie, however, he was only one amongst eight other equally qualified physicians. Each time he attempted to take all responsibility for decision making, one of his peers would intercede. It became obvious that his leadership pattern was not productive in this situation and not to his nor his patient's advantage.

2. Laissez-Faire Leadership

LAISSEZ-FAIRE leadership is based on the premise that non-interference is best. Although a LAISSEZ-FAIRE leader is assigned his leadership position, he is ineffectual in decision making, task assignment, supervision, and completion of tasks. Whereas the AUTHORITARIAN leader makes all the decisions for the group, the LAISSEZ-FAIRE leader doesn't make any decisions. LAISSEZ-FAIRE is French for "let them do as they wish." The LAISSEZ-FAIRE leader leaves all decision to his team. This can produce confusion that results in poorer health care for patients.

Example

The child life program at the hospital is highly necessary for the children's well-being. The program is a new one, however, and is viewed sceptically by many of the traditional staff. The mandate under which the program functions is loose and directed primarily towards recreation. The director of the program has been chosen because of a long commitment to the hospital's volunteer program. She has no more skills in therapeutic assistance for the hospitalized child than most of her staff, and she has little skill in administration. In fact, she becomes anxious that she may be expected to provide clinical expertise. She begins to withdraw. Meetings are held, but they have no agenda and no clear outcome. There are decided discrepancies in staff functioning, and requests for inservice education or increased staff are unmet.

3. Democratic Leadership

DEMOCRATIC leadership ensures that group members have a say in important decision making that affects them. People seem to be more productive when they share a collegial relationship with their co-workers. This interaction is based on mutual respect and minimizes stress on status and hierarchy. The leader can still take ultimate responsbility for the decision, but usually this is based on the culmination of group opinions and problem-solving which has helped the leader to arrive at a better, more informed decision. There also seems to be more job satisfaction and increased quality of care when leadership is DEMOCRATIC rather than AUTHORITARIAN or LAISSEZ-FAIRE.

Example

The head nurse on the ward to which Josie is admitted is notably democratic in her leadership, and this has precipitated her goal of an interdisciplinary sharing in the care of Josie. The head nurse is aware of the difficulties in Josie's care, but she views the difficulties as challenges all staff members can contribute to and problem solve together.

Exercise 48:   Leadership, Role Negotiation, and Conflict

Purpose: To examine leadership, role negotiations, and conflict.

Instructions: Using a group whose members have interacted together before:

1. The group leader assigns each of five persons a role on a health care team (e.g., physician, nurse, etc.). The assigned role is written in large letters on a piece of paper, which is pinned on the shirt of each participant so that other members can see it.

2. The leader reads the following: "In complete silence, the group is to assign themselves in order of importance to the patient."

3. Ten minutes later, the leader calls a halt to the activities and the following questions are examined by the group as a whole.

Questions for Discussion

- How did the group communicate? Who initiated this, and how did the pattern spread?
- Was the assignment accomplished? How did the group determine a priority?
- Did a leader emerge who directed the group? Did the group accept the leadership, or did they assign another leader?
- Did any conflict arise? Was it dealt with? How? Was it resolved?

E. COMMUNICATION

Communication is the transmission of information. In a simple interaction, this may be its only function (e.g., asking for, and receiving, the time). Communication can, however, be very complex since it provides information about situations and relationships. Thus, the team member, interacting with other team members or patients, expresses and receives information which enables or retards the continuation of relationships and functioning within the health care organization.

Communication occurs through a FEEDFORWARD–FEEDBACK method, which looks, diagrammatically, like this:

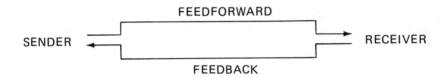

For health professionals, it is important to have access to information that only the patient has. You, as the health professional (SENDER) may ask (FEEDFORWARD) the patient (RECEIVER) the message "How do you feel?" Your feedback may be verbal: "I have the most terrible pain in my hand," or non-verbal: "a frown."

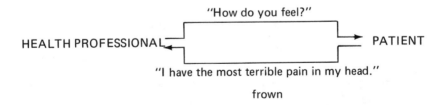

Difficulties arise when the feedforward and feedback are unclear. If the health professional asks, "Well, what's today been like?" meaning "How are you feeling today," but the patient understands the message as "What has the weather been like today?" the health professional may receive an answer far removed from the question he thought he asked.

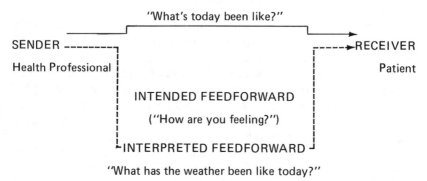

FEEDFORWARD

"What's today been like?"

SENDER ‑ ‑ ‑ ‑ ‑ ‑ ‑ ‑ ‑ ‑ ‑ ‑ ‑ ‑ ‑►RECEIVER

Health Professional   Patient

INTENDED FEEDFORWARD

("How are you feeling?")

INTERPRETED FEEDFORWARD

"What has the weather been like today?"

Therefore, there can be a discrepancy between the intended and interpreted message because of lack of CLARITY in transmission and reception. This can happen in feedforward and feedback.

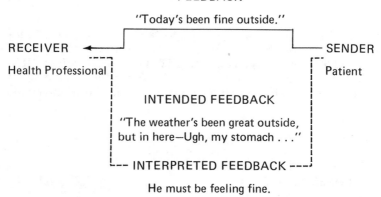

FEEDBACK

"Today's been fine outside."

RECEIVER ◄   SENDER

Health Professional   Patient

INTENDED FEEDBACK

"The weather's been great outside, but in here—Ugh, my stomach . . ."

INTERPRETED FEEDBACK

He must be feeling fine.

Communication and its PERCEPTION are largely dependent on CLARITY and DIRECTION. Clarity refers to how clearly the transmitted message is understood by the sender and receiver. Direction refers to the path of transmission.

Example

Josephine is angry with her doctor.

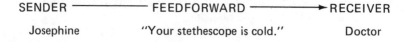

SENDER ───────── FEEDFORWARD ─────────► RECEIVER

Josephine   "Your stethescope is cold."   Doctor

The sender's feedforward, although directed appropriately, is masked or unclear. Although the direction of the message was appropriate, the clarity was not. The doctor must be very perceptive to recognize the intended anger.

Example

Mrs. Jones was angry at the physicians who discuss Josephine's case in the hall just outside Josie's room.

SENDER ─────── FEEDFORWARD ──────────►RECEIVER

Mrs. Jones   "The doctors on the ward make me   Nurse on ward
               angry when they discuss Josie's case
               where she can hear it. I think it frightens
               her. Why can't they discuss that "stuff"
               somewhere else?"

Although the sender's message is clear, it is not directed to the source of the problem. In fact, Mrs. Jones has labelled a concern shared by the nursing staff, who have tried unsuccessfully to deal with the problem. If Mrs. Jones had spoken directly to the involved physicians, they might have been able to explain or alter their behavior.

Example

Mrs. Jones is angry because the diet she had ordered for Josie's lunch had not been sent. Instead, the dietician had chosen a high protein diet, and Mrs. Jones felt Josie would not eat this. Mrs. Jones protested to another mother.

SENDER──────── FEEDFORWARD ──────────►RECEIVER

Mrs. Jones   "I don't think any of them want Josie   Another mother
               to have what she wants."

The message is directed inappropriately since the other mother is in no position to refute or condone the remark, and the message itself is so unclear that action is difficult to initiate.

Another important component of communication is who sends and who receives. The same feedforward might elicit two very different responses depending on the sender. We might respond to the question, "What have you been doing today?" with one answer for a neighbor ("Oh, just working.") and another for a colleague relieving us on evening shift ("Three lumbar punctures and two bone marrows."). Communication, therefore, defines the nature of the relationship between the interactants in the organization.

Communication can also control by functioning as a system of mutual regulation of behavior between people.

Example

Shortly after Josephine's admission, Dr. Brown noted that her calcium imbalance made her a prime risk for tetany. He suggested that all resources should be directed to correcting the imbalance. Josie's labile electrolyte balance and the energy directed towards it was frightening for the child life staff who provided recreational alternatives for the children. They were anxious not to have Josie in the playroom without nurses and physicians present. Since this was impossible, the child life staff voiced their reluctance to participate in interactions with Josie in the playroom.

By placing a heavy emphasis on written and oral communication on Josie's electrolyte situation, Dr. Brown had made that almost the sole focus of activity of the ward staff. In this situation, communication by way of non-communication (ie., no explanation of tetany or its physical manifestations and management) caused the child life staff as a group to withdraw from activities with Josie.

Communication occurs continuously. It is, in fact, impossible not to communicate. Even silence conveys a message.

Example

A conference was held to organize and coordinate the activities related to Josie's heart surgery. During the meeting, someone asked, "Is there a primary nurse involved in Josie's care?" There was no answer. The question was then asked, "Are any of the nurses interested in volunteering to be Josie's primary nurse?" Again there was silence. All present at the meeting interpreted the silence as refusal.

To communicate, man relies heavily on the spoken and written word. Language is learned. Newborns quickly learn to express their dissatisfactions and needs by crying. Parents learn to differentiate these cries and respond accordingly. As the child grows, he or she masters language, and others begin to expect the child to respond with language rather than by crying and pointing.

Example

Josie had learned that, by crying and screaming, she was able to obtain what she wanted. When she wanted candy rather than vegetables, she often screamed at her mother and the staff, and this usually elicited the desired results for her. Her behavior had, however, produced anger and frustration in the staff and was a reason why no one would volunteer to be primarily involved in Josie's care.

By instituting, with the mother's co-operation, a behavior modification program, it was possible to encourage Josie to use language to produce the desired results. The staff, by ignoring her shrill attention-seeking cries, extinguished this behavior. The staff, as a team, had specifically communicated to Josie that her method of communication was unacceptable and would be unprofitable for her.

Most messages are conveyed through multiple channels. The channels may enhance or contradict the basic verbal message. It is, therefore, important to recognize all forms of feedforward and feedback.

Example

As the behavior modification program began, Josie quickly recognized that her cries and shrill orders to the staff were not eliciting the desired results. The staff then became aware that, although Josie's shrill condemnations and cries to "Get out" were still taking place, her finger would curl beckoningly for staff members to stay with her.

Similarly, for all children on Josie's ward, the presence of the intravenous therapy team, which was responsible for starting new intravenous lines, elicited fear, passivity, and general apathy. The children, Josie included, recognized that, until the team left the ward,

any one of them could be the recipient of an intravenous needle. Protest would be useless.

Communication, whether verbal or non-verbal, transmits
messages about content and relationships between people and
among organizations. Understanding the function of communication is vital to the understanding of teams and organizations.

Exercise 49:   Communication Patterns

Purpose: To examine communication patterns in a small
group.

Instructions: 1.   The group leader divides the group into small
groups of six persons.

2.   One person in the group is assigned the role of
"observer." The observer is to draw the pattern of communications as they occur. This
is done by first drawing small circles on a
piece of paper to represent each of the five
members.

Each time one member talks to another,
the observer should draw a line on his paper
from the speaker to the person spoken to.
Each time a speaker speaks to the group as a
whole, a line should be drawn from the speaker
to the letters GP.

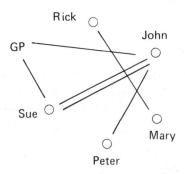

3.   The groups are given ten minutes to discuss
the topic "Euthanasia—Does the patient have
a say in his own demise?" The observer records the interaction pattern.

4. After ten minutes, the group stops and examines the "sociogram" drawn by the observer.

Questions for Discussion

- Did one person dominate the conversation more than any other?
- Did any two persons participate more than any others? Why?
- Did any one person participate less than any others? Why?
- Did any off-topic conversations begin? How was this handled?
- Did any person emerge as a leader or organizer of the discussion? How did this person achieve that role?

5. Have the group resume the conversation for an additional ten minutes. This time the group should strive to ensure that everyone has equal chance to talk. The observer again records group interaction. After ten minutes, the observer gives the group feedback.

Questions for Discussion

- Did the participation rate in the group change as a result of the initial feedback?
- What are the advantages and disadvantages of ensuring that everyone in the group gets a chance to participate?

F. CLIMATE

The climate or atmosphere in which the organization functions is important for the accomplishment of the goals. The goals can best be accomplished if there is a unity and cohesiveness within the organization that allows for individual differences yet draws the members together so that a common approach can be presented.

The cohesive climate is dependent on norms and values of the organization being examined and clarified and differences tolerated so that work can be accomplished.

Example

One month had gone by, and the staff were still focused primarily on Josie's electrolyte imbalance. No mention had been made of when the problems Mrs. Jones saw as vital to her daughter's recovery would be dealt with. When she questioned the staff, they seemed unresponsive. She began to doubt their ability, and her trust in Dr. Brown decreased. She became more symbiotic in her relationship with Josie, and this aggravated Josie's sick role behavior. This frustrated the staff, who began to avoid the mother and child, and the problem was further aggravated. The staff began to see the work they had done with this family disintegrating. This caused them to doubt their own abilities. It was crucial that the head nurse and Dr. Brown intervene to alter the situation and thus alter the climate of distrust and anxiety that had developed.

G. CONFLICT

Conflict occurs when values or goals are incompatible. It is a kind of opposition directed at the perceived obstacle.

Example

Josephine's major medical problems necessitated prolonged hospitalization—five months in her own community and a month in the specialty hospital. Very legitimate fears for her life have been voiced during the entire period. Mrs. Jones and many of the health professionals have responded to this fear by cajoling and coercing Josie into participating in her treatments and other interactions. Josie has become very skilled at manipulating situations to her advantage. By maintaining and exploiting the sick role, she obtains many toys and treats that are important to her self-esteem. She also avoids many painful and frightening situations.

The staff members have a variety of responses to Josie's behavior. Some think it entirely appropriate and a healthy way of coping with prolonged hospitalization and life-threatening anomalies. Others, however, see Josie's behavior as a function of parental and staff discomfort with Josie's situation. They are concerned by the amount of control that Josie has and her seeming inability to relax and be a child with others in control.

The discrepant perceptions produced major conflicts on the ward. There was no common approach to Josie, and this further aggravated her behavior.

Conflict performs important functions for the organization (Jandt, 1969). It establishes group boundaries by strengthening group cohesiveness and affirming separateness. It decreases tension by bringing underlying conflict out into the open. Resolved conflict can clarify objectives and establish group norms.

Example

The situation became explosive one day when Josie refused to attend the hospital school program. Although this was not a compulsory program for any hospitalized child, regular attendance was encouraged for those children who were able to go. Two staff members became embroiled in a heated discussion abouth whether Josie should or should not attend school. The ward staff quickly organized themselves. Those who felt Josie ought to have her own way felt she could decide about school. Those who felt the adults on the ward should execute some control in the situation felt that the staff and the mother should be responsible for the school attendance decision, not Josie. The heated discussion brought the conflicting opinions out in the open and allowed the head nurse to intercede to resolve the conflict.

Management of the above conflict could produce the following results:

Response by Group or Leader	Effect on Task
1. Smoothing over, ignoring the real problem.	not accomplished well
2. Forcing a solution through use of authority	may be accomplished
3. Compromise	may be accomplished
4. Confrontation	not accomplished initially then accomplished very well

Example

The head nurse called a patient care meeting. Using the confrontation approach, she labelled the problem which had precipitated the discussion. She then pushed the staff to take the problem one step further and determine what were the basic differences in their approach to paediatric care. This forced the staff to examine their discrepant values and eventually, through much discussion and soul-searching, to develop a solid approach to Josie's care. The staff were, in future, much more cognizant of the child's needs, her stage of emotional and physical development, and their role in furthering Josie's healthy development.

SUMMARY

Groups, teams, and organizations are important to health professionals because of the way in which health care is provided. Factors such as goals, roles, leadership, authority, climate, communication, and conflict are crucial to the health professional's understanding of organizational function.

9
Developing Skills in Assessing Interpersonal Skills

A. THE IMPORTANCE OF ASSESSING INTERPERSONAL SKILLS

There are five main reasons why health professionals are interested in assessing interpersonal skills:

1. Instructors assess their students' interpersonal skills in order to determine students' strongest and weakest interpersonal skills. Particular educational programs may require that students demonstrate minimal competency in specific interpersonal skills. In order to assess whether a student has attained minimal competency in an interpersonal skill, it is essential to measure in some way the student's demonstration of that skill. Instructors may assess students' interpersonal skills for the purpose of grading for a course in which interpersonal skills are taught. Instructors may also assess students' interpersonal skills prior to a course in order to determine the particular learning needs of students. For example, a student who scores low on FACILITATION skills but high on PROBLEM-SOLVING skills will need to concentrate on learning FACILITATION SKILLS. Assessment not only identifies the student's weakest skills, it also provides a baseline measure against which any improvement in the specific interpersonal skills can be compared. By assessing a student's interpersonal skills before and after instruction, it is possible to determine how much the student has improved. This is valuable feedback for both instructor and student.

2. Instructors use assessment of students' interpersonal skills as a means of assessing the quality of the educational programs used to teach interpersonal skills. By comparing gains in student scores (from pre- to post-assessment) and by comparing student scores for different classes and even different years (in which the course is taught), instructors can get an idea of how effective their teaching is. One of the key questions every instructor must ask himself is: Did my students learn anything? When students fail to learn an interpersonal skill, the deficit may be in the teacher, or the educational program, rather than in the student. Assessment of interpersonal skills provides important feedback for instructors.

3. Health professional learners assess their own interpersonal skills in order to keep their interpersonal skills sharp and in order to search for ways of improving their responses to specific situations with patients or other health professionals. There are many practicing health professionals who believe in this type of self-

directed learning. They take the initiative to self-assess, or to have their peers assess, their interviewing and interpersonal skills on a regular basis. This assessment may be as informal as having a colleague listen to an audiotape the health professional has made of a patient interview, or it may be as formal as having several colleagues rate a videotape the health professional has made of a patient interview.

4. Educational programs use assessment of prospective students' interpersonal skills as a means of screening for suitable candidates for their programs. This is an admissions screening procedure. At a well-known health professional school, a case recently occurred where a third-year student demonstrated excellence in his clinical skills but failed to demonstrate minimal competence in his interpersonal skills. The student refused to take remedial interpersonal skills training and was subsequently dropped from the program. This is the sort of problem that admissions assessment of prospective students' interpersonal skills is designed to prevent.

5. Researchers assess the interpersonal skills of health professionals in order to determine the effects of specific interpersonal skills on patients. At McMaster University in Hamilton, Canada, Dr. Peter Tugwell is the principal investigator of a current study investigating the relationship between the process of health care given to myocardial infarction patients and patient outcome. One of the process variables being assessed is the interpersonal skills the physician uses with his or her myocardial infarction patients. In the last decade, there has been a sharp increase in the number of studies done on quality of care assessment (much of them based on measurement of clinical records). This interest in the assessment of clinical care is now being paralleled by a similar interest and growth in the area of assessment of health professionals' interpersonal skills.

The main obstacle to health professionals learning to assess their interpersonal skills is anxiety about being evaluated. The technical term for this is evaluation anxiety—fear of being negatively evaluated. Some health professionals (whether students or practitioners) are afraid that if their interpersonal skills are assessed, they will score poorly. Because criticism or making mistakes is a stressor for them, they try to avoid being assessed to avoid experiencing stress. This is a common response to being assessed, and one not unique to health professionals. Having your interpersonal skills assessed can provide you with valuable information about your strengths and weaknesses. For this reason it is important that you be aware of any feelings about being assessed that you might have that could prevent you from actively involving yourself in the assessment process. If your interpersonal skills are weak in one area, having your interpersonal skills measured will provide you with valuable feedback on what that area is. Many health professionals are not clearly aware of what their strong and their weak interpersonal skills are. Assessment provides you with corrective feedback—information about your skill level that you can use to improve your interpersonal skills. Can you accept negative feedback about your interpersonal skills? It's important that you can. If you need to improve your skills in a particular area, it is essential that you allow yourself to notice and to accept that you do need improvement. There is a quote attributed to the psychiatrist Rudolf Driekurs that sums up the sort of attitude health professionals need to take to learn from having their interpersonal skills assessed. The quote is: "Adults need the courage to be imperfect." Having your interpersonal skills measured and assessed can help you to become a more effective health professional.

If you have been practicing the interpersonal skills presented in this book, you may be wondering how well you are doing. This chapter tells you how to assess your interpersonal skills in a number of ways so that you can receive clear feedback on your present level of competence. You will also learn how to assess the interpersonal skills of your peers and colleagues so that you can give them feedback on their interpersonal skills and help them to become more effective health professionals.

B. ISSUES IN ASSESSING INTERPERSONAL SKILLS

There are six important issues that must be considered when assessing interpersonal skills. They are:

1. What interpersonal skills should be assessed?
2. How should interpersonal skills be measured?
3. In what type of situation should interpersonal skills be assessed?
4. Who should assess interpersonal skills?
5. How is the reliability of the assessment method to be determined?
6. Is the assessment method valid?

Each of these important issues is discussed in detail below.

1. What Interpersonal Skills Should Be Assessed?

Once you decide to assess your own or someone else's interpersonal skills, the first consideration is to determine which specific interpersonal skills you are going to assess. There are too many different interpersonal skills to assess at one time, so some limiting decision must be made. The experimental and theoretical literature on interpersonal skills suggests that at least four different interpersonal skills should be assessed for health professionals. They are: WARMTH, ACTIVE LISTENING (also known as empathy), ASSERTIVENESS, and INITIATING.

WARMTH and ACTIVE LISTENING are relevant because of the experimental evidence that indicates these FACILITATION skills produce a variety of physiological, psychological, and behavioral outcomes for patients (Gerrard, 1978). ASSERTIVENESS is an important skill for health professionals to assess because it is an interpersonal skill useful for handling aggressive patients and team conflict—two problem areas frequently encountered by health professionals. Whereas WARMTH and ACTIVE LISTENING are basically trust-building skills, INITIATING is a task and problem-oriented interpersonal skill. Health professionals use INITIATING to encourage the patient to take some action that will help the patient solve his problem. INITIATING includes: giving information, carrying out some physical action, initiating a discussion, offering an alternative solution, making requests, and stating an opinion. INITIATING includes the action and task-oriented interpersonal skills described in the behavior change and problem-solving chapters.

These interpersonal skills relate to a two-stage model of helping. The first stage is one of building rapport; the second stage is one of taking action. You help the patient to trust you, then you get him (if necessary) to take some action that will help him get well. First you FACILITATE, then you INITIATE ACTION. In actual practice these two stages may overlap. The main idea, however, is that both skills are important and that each has a different goal. ASSERTIVENESS relates to the two primary interpersonal skills of FACILITATION and INITIATING in that it is a conflict reducing skill that may be employed in either the FACILITATION or the INITIATING "phase" of the interview.

2. How Should Interpersonal Skills Be Measured?

There are three main ways of measuring interpersonal skills—each having its particular advantages and disadvantages:

    a) Written feedback.

    b) Rating scales.

    c) Content analysis.

Written feedback. This form of measurement is the simplest way to assess interpersonal skills. While you observe a health professional conduct an interview with a patient, you simply write down examples of good and of poor interpersonal skills as they occur during the interview.

Example

Jim, a health professional student, is observing Ann, another health professional student, conduct an interview with a patient. Jim is in another room and observes the interview through a one-way mirror. Some of Jim's observations of Ann's interpersonal skills are recorded on the following sheet.

WRITTEN FEEDBACK OBSERVATION SHEET   Date: October 5

Interviewer: Ann

Observer: Jim

Time	Positive Behavior	Room for Improvement
1	Ann introduces herself and says hello; seems confident.	
2	Smiles at patient, invites questions (initiates).	Folds her arms—closed posture.
3	(Patient is talking.)	Leans away from the patient. Ann seems a little nervous.
4	Reflects patient's feelings. "You're really worried about that."	Misses content of patient's speech.
5	(Patient is talking)	
6		"Don't be afraid"—poor active listening—shuts off patient's feelings.
7	Warm voice tone.	
8	Good initiating: "Could we talk about this a little more?"	
9	(Patient is talking.)	
10	Gives patient some appropriate information (good initiating).	
11	Gives patient information and suggests alternative solution to patient's problem.	Patient has puzzled look on face—Ann didn't pick up on this.
12	Mentions patient's name as she closes interview, shakes patient's hand.	

This observation sheet has time intervals recorded on the left hand side. The numbers correspond to the number of minutes (approximate) that have elapsed since the start of the interview.

When Jim gives Ann feedback on her interview, he will be able to give her a rough idea when during the interview a specific behavior he recorded occurred. Two types of observations are made: "Positive Behavior," which refers to the use of good interpersonal skills, and "Room for Improvement," under which the use of poor interpersonal skills is noted. The main advantages of written feedback are that it requires no special training to use and it provides useful, specific information for the person receiving the feedback. Instead of being told that her overall level of ACTIVE LISTENING was 3.0 (out of a possible 4.0), Ann can be given specific information on what she actually said or failed to say. Students find this sort of specific feedback very helpful. The main disadvantage of written feedback is that it is not quantifiable. This means that the overall skill level of the person being assessed is not identified in precise terms. In order to compare Ann's performance with those of other students—or even herself at a later time—translating her performance into a meaningful score is desirable. Written feedback is too imprecise to allow this. When precise measurement is required, as in research on interpersonal skills, written feedback should not be used. Although students appreciate the specific information they receive in written feedback, its imprecision makes it inadequate for meaningful pre/post assessment, evaluation of program effectiveness, comparison of students, or research purposes. Nevertheless, written feedback is useful because of its specific nature.

Exercise 50:   Written Feedback

Purpose: To develop skills in giving and receiving written feedback on interpersonal skills.

Instructions: 1. Divide the group into small groups of four.

2. Each group member makes a 10-minute videotape of himself interviewing a patient.

3. Each small group meets and views the videotapes made by its members. As each group member shows his videotape, the other group members should use the Observation Sheet provided to give written feedback to the "interviewer." (Xerox the Observation Sheet so that you will have a copy for each member of your small group; or copy the Observation Sheet headings onto separate pieces of paper, one for each member of your small group.)

As you observe each videotape, try to provide written feedback on the interviewer's use of ACTIVE LISTENING, WARMTH (particularly his non-verbal behavior) and INITIATING. Write down examples of what he actually said and did. The more specific you can be about the behavior you observed, the more valuable your feedback will be for the "interviewer."

If you do not have access to videotape recording and playback equipment, observe an actual interview through a one-way mirror in an interviewing observation room, or listen to audio-tapes made of actual patient interviews made by group members. Videotaping your interview is ideal because it permits you to "go back" and check out "what actually occurred."

Questions for Discussion

- Did the rest of your group point out similar "Positive" and "Room for Improvement" behaviors that they noticed in your interview? That is, how strongly did the group agree about how well you conducted your interview?
- Did you agree with the feedback you received?

WRITTEN FEEDBACK OBSERVATION SHEET	Date: _____
	Interviewer: _____
	Observer: _____

Time	Positive Behavior	Room for Improvement
1		
2		
3		
4		
5		
6		
7		
8		
9		
10		

Rating Scales.   A scale is a measuring device that is used to assign numbers to behaviors according to predetermined rules. Rating scales are a widely used method for measuring interpersonal skills.

One of the simplest types of rating scales is the Semantic-Differential. It consists of a pair of polar adjectives or phrases separated by a series of undefined scale positions. For example:

WARM   ____ ____ ____ ____ ____ ____ ____   COLD

To use the Semantic-Differential rating scale, you place a check mark closest to the adjective that describes the behavior of the person you are observing. In the previous example, Jim found Ann's interviewing behavior to be moderately warm, so his rating for Ann would look like this:

WARM   ____ _√__ ____ ____ ____ ____ ____   COLD

Once a rater has checked off a space on the Semantic-Differential, a number can be assigned to each scale position.

```
        4.0   3.5   3.0   2.5   2.0   1.5   1.0
```
WARM   ____ _√__ ____ ____ ____ ____ ____   COLD

The warmth rating that Jim assigned to Ann is 3.5 out of a possible 4.0. Translating the checked position on the scale to a number facilitates recording, statistical analysis, and student feedback. If a student is rated for WARMTH before and after a course in interpersonal skills, he can be given feedback on his performance in the form of numbers. For example: "In your interviews before the course your average WARMTH score was 2.0; after the course your WARMTH score averaged 3.5."

The Likert scale is somewhat similar to the Semantic-Differential scale. It consists of a) a statement about the interviewer's behavior, and b) to the right of the statement, several scale positions representing varying degrees of agreement and disagreement with the statement. For example,

The health professional was WARM.   SA (MA) SLA IB SLD MD SD

SA	=	Strongly Agree
MA	=	Moderately Agree
SLA	=	Slightly Agree
IB	=	In Between
SLD	=	Slightly Disagree
MD	=	Moderately Disagree
SD	=	Strongly Disagree

To use the Likert scale you circle the letters that represent the extent to which you agree with the statement you are considering. If there are several statements to be rated, the abbreviations (SA, MA, etc.) can be repeated beside each statement. Alternatively, columns representing each category of agreement can be drawn so that the rater can indicate his agreement with each statement by placing a check mark in the appropriate column.

	4.0	3.5	3.0	2.5	2.0	1.5	1.0
	SA	MA	SLA	IB	SLD	MD	SD
1. The health professional was WARM		√					
2. The health professional used ACTIVE LISTENING			√				
3. The health professional INITIATED			√				

The Likert scale can be scored similar to the Semantic-Differential scale by assigning numbers to each scale position.

The main disadvantage of the Semantic-Differential and Likert rating scales is that their scale points are not well-defined. If Jim assesses Ann's WARMTH as 3.5 on the Semantic-Differential or Likert scale, what exactly does that mean in behavioral terms? We don't know because each scale point is not precisely defined. A rater who has friends who rarely express WARMTH openly may "strongly agree" that Ann is WARM in her interview. A second rater, whose friends are *very* WARM, may only "slightly agree" that Ann is WARM. When scale positions are undefined, each rater will impose (usually unconsciously) his own definition of what each scale position means. When scale positions are not explicitly defined, it is easy for raters to disagree about what they see.

The problem of undefined scale positions is overcome by the behaviorally anchored rating scale. This is a rating scale that has each scale position described in terms of specific behavior. If the behavior observed matches the behavior description for the scale position, then that scale position is the correct one. Each scale position is "anchored" by explicit descriptions of interviewer behavior that fit that scale position. This makes ratings somewhat more objective since raters are now using a common set of definitions for each scale position. Behaviorally anchored rating scales for ACTIVE LISTENING (also called EMPATHY), WARMTH,

ASSERTIVENESS, and INITIATING are shown on the following pages. Although behavioral descriptions are only given for four scale points (1.0, 2.0, 3.0, and 4.0), you can use the mid-points on the scale when you are rating someone's behavior. Each scale has seven different rating points (i.e., 1.0, 1.5, 2.0, 2.5, 3.0, 3.5, 4.0).

Level 3.0 is generally considered to be the level of minimal competence in the interpersonal skill being assessed. That is, if you obtain a score of 3.0 in ACTIVE LISTENING, then you have demonstrated—in the interview for which you are being assessed—minimal competence in ACTIVE LISTENING. It is not uncommon for most health professional students to score 1.5 to 2.0 on these rating scales before being trained in interpersonal skills. Examples of different rating scales follow.

Example

A patient says: "This pain just doesn't seem to go away. No matter what I try, it's still there. I just don't know what I'm going to do.

RATING SCALE FOR ACTIVE LISTENING (EMPATHY)

Rating	General Description of Scale Position	Behavioral Description of Scale Position	Sample Health Professional Responses
4.0	Very good response	Underlying feelings and content are accurately reflected.	"You're afraid because you think you might not get better and you don't know what to do to help yourself."
3.0	Good response	Surface feelings and content are accurately reflected.	"You're worried because you're sick so much."
2.0	Poor response	Content only is reflected.	"You think your illness isn't going to go away."
1.0	Very poor response	Neither feeling nor content is reflected. Presence of subtractive element (a destructive response)	"I'd like to take your blood pressure now. Roll up your sleeve please." "Don't be silly. Of course you're going to get better."

272

Example

A health professional is meeting a female patient, age 43, for the first time.

RATING SCALE FOR WARMTH

Rating	General Description of Scale Position	Behavioral Description of Scale Position	Sample Health Professional Responses
4.0	Very good response	Very warm voice tone; relaxed posture; face, posture and behavior show marked interest and attentiveness; behavior and speech content show deep respect and consideration for the other person. Very friendly behavior.	The health professional smiles, walks over to the patient, warmly says, "Hello, Mrs. Jones, my name is Bill Smith," and shakes her hand. The health professional sits down, leans slightly toward the patient, maintains eye contact with the patient, and says, "What seems to be the problem?"
3.0	Good response	Warm voice tone; relaxed posture; face and posture show interest and attentiveness; behavior and speech content show respect and consideration for the other person. Friendly behavior.	The health professional walks over to the patient and says, "Hello, Mrs. Jones, my name is Bill Smith." The health professional sits down, leans slightly forward, and says, "What seems to be the problem?"
2.0	Poor response	Slightly cool voice tone; slightly tense posture; face and posture show indifference; behavior and speech content convey slight disinterest in the other person. Slightly unfriendly behavior.	The health professional walks over to the patient and says, "I'm Dr. Smith." The health professional sits down, avoids looking at the patient for several seconds while he shuffles through some papers. He looks up, a slightly bored expression on his face, and he says, "What seems to be the problem?"
1.0	Very poor response	Very cold voice tone; tense posture; face and posture show disinterest; behavior and speech content show disregard for the other person. Very unfriendly behavior.	The health professional walks over to the patient and, still standing, says, "What's your problem?" His arms are folded across his chest, his voice is cold, and he looks as though he is in a hurry.

Example

A patient says: "This pain just doesn't seem to go away. No matter what I try, it's still there. I just don't know what I'm going to do."

RATING SCALE FOR INITIATING

Rating	General Description of Scale Position	Behavioral Description of Scale Position	Sample Health Professional Responses
4.0	Very good response	Invites the other person to talk further.	"Where exactly are you hurting?"
3.0	Good response	Shows one of the following responses: a) Offers alternative solution. b) Initiates appropriate physical action.	"I want to check your blood pressure. Roll up your sleeve please."
2.0	Poor response	Gives appropriate information only.	"Once we find out what kind of pain you're having, then we'll be able to help you."
1.0	Very poor response	A very inappropriate initiating response, or the complete absence of an initiating response.	"I can't help you—I'm just a student."

Example

A male patient, age 63, says, "Since my heart attack my wife has been treating me like a baby. She does everything for me—even things I can do myself. But I must say, the pain is gone and I rarely need the nitroglycerine tablets".

RATING SCALE FOR INITIATING (Continued)

Rating	General Description of Scale Position	Behavioral Description of Scale Position	Sample Health Professional Responses
4.0	Very good response	Invites the other person to talk further.	"You sound pretty upset about the way your wife's been treating you. Could we talk about this a bit more?"
3.0	Good response	Shows one of the following responses: a) Offers alternative solution. b) Initiates appropriate physical action.	"Perhaps you could bring your wife in on your next visit, and we'll reassure her and talk to her about the importance of letting you be more independent."
2.0	Poor response	Gives appropriate information.	"Your wife is acting the way many wives do when their husbands have heart attacks. She's probably afraid that if you exert yourself, you'll have another heart attack."
1.0	Very poor response	A very inappropriate initiating response, or the complete absence of an initiating response.	"I'm glad to hear the pain is gone."

Example

A health professional has a full morning of patients booked. Mr. Thomas' 5-year-old daughter was scheduled for a ten-minute appointment to have stitches removed from her chin. After they were removed, Mr. Thomas handed the health professional a lengthy school physical form and said: "Could you take care of this as well? It would save me a second trip?"

RATING SCALE FOR ASSERTIVENESS

Rating	General Description of Scale Position	Behavioral Description of Scale Position	Sample Health Professional Response
4.0	Very good response	Displays a high level of confidence; refuses unreasonable request or points out put-down without hesitating or apologizing; shows no anxiety; voice tone is firm, confident.	"I would like to be able to save you a second trip, but we only scheduled a ten-minute appointment today for removal of stitches. Completing that form requires taking a more complete physical examination. I have other patients waiting to be seen, so it will not be possible to do it today. My secretary will be happy to schedule a time for next week."
3.0	Good response	Refuses unreasonable request; points out put-down; may show slight hesitation.	"Oh. . .uh. . .I'd like to do it but we only scheduled a ten-minute appointment today for removal of stitches. Uh. . .I have. . .uh. . .other patients waiting to be seen so it will not be possible to do it today. My secretary will be happy to schedule a time for next week."
2.0	Poor response	Fails to refuse unreasonable request; ignores verbal attack; acts anxious and defensive; attacks or blames other person.	"Oh (slight pause). . .alright."
1.0	Very poor response	No response; acts very anxious, sub-missive, defensive, or aggressive; gives in to unreasonable request.	"Uh. . .er. . .uh. . .let's see (looks at the form). . .well, alright (has angry look on face)." "You've got a lot of nerve. Can't you see I have other patients? Come back next week."

Exercise 51:   Rating Interpersonal Skills

Purpose: To develop skills in rating interpersonal skills.

Instructions: 1. Divide the class into small groups of 6 to 8 persons.

2. Each group member makes a 10-minute video-tape of himself interviewing a patient.

3. Each small group views and rates each video-tape made by its members using the behaviorally anchored rating scales for ACTIVE LISTENING, WARMTH, INITIATING, and ASSERTIVENESS.

Use the attached Interpersonal Skills Rating Form to rate each videotape (xerox additional forms so that you have one feedback form for each group member). At one-minute intervals, rate the interviewer on all four interpersonal skills. If you feel that one of the interpersonal skills does not apply to the one-minute segment you are rating, write NA (for not applicable). For example, if during a one-minute segment the patient does all the talking, it is not meaningful to rate the interviewer on ACTIVE LISTENING or INITIATING (although he could be rated on non-verbal behavior for WARMTH and ASSERTIVENESS). If the interview lasts longer than ten minutes, make your ratings for additional one-minute segments in the spaces provided.

4. To score the rating form, add together your scores for each interpersonal skill and write the total in the space provided. Divide by the total number of ratings you made for that interpersonal skill, and write the average or mean ($\bar{x}$) score in the space provided. This scoring procedure is illustrated on the Interpersonal Skills Rating Form shown, which has been scored for the example of Ann (see section on written feedback). The "Positive" and "Room For Improvement" behaviors described on the Written Feedback Observation Sheet have been

treated as representative of the health professional's behavior during each one-minute segment of her interview and assigned scores from the behaviorally anchored scales.

EXAMPLE: INTERPERSONAL SKILLS RATING FORM

Date: ___October___

Interviewer: ___Ann___

Rater: ___Jim___

Time (Minutes)	Active Listening	Warmth	Initiating	Assertiveness
1	NA	3.5	NA	3.0
2	NA	3.5	3.0	2.5
3	NA	2.0	NA	1.5
4	2.5	3.0	NA	2.5
5	NA	3.0	NA	3.0
6	1.0	3.5	NA	3.0
7	3.0	3.5	NA	3.0
8	NA	3.0	3.0	3.5
9	NA	3.0	NA	3.0
10	NA	3.0	2.5	3.0
11	2.0	3.0	NA	3.0
12	NA	3.5	NA	3.0
13				
14				
15				
Total	8.5	37.5	12.5	34.0
Divide by	4	12	4	14
Average	2.1	3.1	3.1	2.8

As can be seen from the ratings, Ann received average scores of 3.1 on both WARMTH and INITIATING. Since 3.0 is indicative of minimal competence, we can assume that Ann is functioning at minimal competence on WARMTH and INITIATING in this interview. Ann's average ASSERTIVENESS score is 2.8, which is quite good. Her nervousness during interview segments 2, 3, and 4 pulled

INTERPERSONAL SKILLS RATING FORM

Date: _____

Interviewer: _____

Rater: _____

Time (Minutes)	Active Listening	Warmth	Initiating	Assertiveness
1				
2				
3				
4				
5				
6				
7				
8				
9				
10				
11				
12				
13				
14				
15				
Total				
Divide by				
Average				

her overall ASSERTIVENESS score down. Ann's average ACTIVE LISTENING score of 2.1 indicates that this is her weakest interpersonal skill—one she needs to improve.

> 5. After each videotape is rated and scored, the group should give the "interviewer" feedback in the form of average scores for each interpersonal skill.

Questions for Discussion

- Do you agree with the feedback scores you received from the rest of the group?
- What was your strongest interpersonal skill? Your weakest interpersonal skill?
- Which interpersonal skill did you have the most difficulty rating? What do you think is the reason for this?

Content analysis. This is a method for counting the frequency with which specific interviewer behaviors occur. When you use a rating scale, you make a judgment about the degree to which an interpersonal skill is present. For example, you decide whether the interviewer's WARMTH skills are very good, good, poor, or very poor (4.0, 3.0, 2.0, or 1.0). You make this judgment on the basis of the extent to which predetermined interviewer WARMTH behaviors are present. You must make a judgment about the quality of the WARMTH present. When you use the content analysis method of assessing interpersonal skills, however, you do not assess the degree to which an interpersonal skill is present. Instead of making a global rating on an interpersonal skill, you simply note the presence or absence of specific behaviors. All you have to decide is: is the behavior there or not?

The Interpersonal Skills Content Analysis Form on the next page illustrates a content analysis scheme for noting the presence/absence of specific behaviors that "make up" each of the interpersonal skills: ACTIVE LISTENING, WARMTH, RESPECT, INITIATING, and ASSERTIVENESS. WARMTH is made up of 18 different specific behaviors. At any one time, a health professional will use several—but not all—of these behaviors to show WARMTH for his patients. The value of such a content analysis system lies in its detail. When you tell a health professional that his behavior with a patient lacked WARMTH, you can identify for him the exact behaviors that were, or were not, present. This type of specific feedback is very useful for the health professional student since it helps him to identify the exact behaviors he needs to change to become more WARM.

The main disadvantage of using content analysis to assess interpersonal skills is that it increases the number of categories an observer must keep track of. Instead of rating a student on four or five interpersonal skills, an observer must now monitor (say) thirty-nine different behaviors. This is a difficult task for any observer and may require the use of multiple observers. Another disadvantage is that sometimes it is the particular combination of two or more interviewer behaviors that produces a positive effect on the patient. An observer using a rating scale might identify this combination of behaviors that results in a level 3.0 rating on WARMTH, whereas an observer using a content analysis scale will not be able to "put the behaviors together" so easily. The fact that one interviewer has many WARMTH behaviors checked off on his form does not necessarily mean that his WARMTH skills are greater than those of an interviewer who has only a few WARMTH behaviors checked off. Which WARMTH behaviors are checked off—in which combination—may make a qualitative difference.

Exercise 52: Assessing Interpersonal Skills Through Content Analysis

Purpose: To develop skills in content analyzing specific interviewer behaviors.

Instructions: 1. Divide the class into small groups of 7.

2. Have each group member prepare a videotape of a 10–15 minute interview with a patient.

3. Each small group meets separately to evaluate its videotapes. As each group member shows his videotape to the small group, the rest of the group members content analyze the interviewer behaviors on the videotape. To reduce the number of behaviors each group member must observe, the following division of content analysis categories is recommended.

Group member	Content Analysis Categories Observed
1	Shows videotape
2	1–3 (these are difficult to score)
3	4–14 (4, 5, 6, and 8 are "once only" behaviors).
4	15–21
5	22–27
6	28–32
7	33–39

INTERPERSONAL SKILLS CONTENT ANALYSIS FORM

Date: _____

Interviewer: _____

Rater: _____

Instructions: Place a tally mark in the column of the appropriate row for each time a behavior is observed.

Behavior	Total
Active Listening	
1. Reflects patient's surface feeling	
2. Reflects patient's underlying feeling	
3. Reflects reason for patient's feeling	
Warmth	
4. Greets patient	
5. Introduces self	
6. Shakes patient's hand	
7. Uses patient's first name	
8. Says goodbye to patient	
9. Maintains eye contact	
10. Faces patient "squarely"	
11. Leans forward slightly	
12. Open posture: arms	
13. Open posture: legs	
14. Relaxed posture	
15. Nods head to show interest	
16. Smiles	
17. Jokes	
18. Talks about patient's "back home" interests	
19. Warm voice tone	
20. Face shows interest, attentiveness	
21. Speech content shows interest	

Behavior	Total
Respect	
22. Answers patient's question	
23. Does not answer patient's question	
24. Fulfills patient's reasonable request	
25. Does not fulfill patient's reasonable request	
26. Health professional invites requests	
27. Tells patient when next interview will be	
Initiating	
28. Gives information	
29. Initiates appropriate discussion of feelings	
30. Initiates appropriate history-taking	
31. Offers alternative solution to problem	
32. Initiates appropriate physical action	
Assertiveness	
33. Fails to refuse unreasonable request	
34. Speech stammers	
35. Hand tremors	
36. Tense facial expression	
37. Touches back of the neck with hand	
38. "Nervous" hand movements	
39. Ignores verbal attack made by patient	

4. After each tape has been viewed and scored, the group members should share with the "interviewer" the total number of times each behavior they observed occurred.

5. Repeat this exercise after the group has received further training in interpersonal skills.

Alternative way of doing this exercise: Select from the Interpersonal Skills Content Analysis Form 6–10 behaviors of most interest to you, (e.g., 2, 3, 9, 16, 19, 26, 29, 30, 34, 36, etc.). Or, assess videotapes on only *one* interpersonal skill dimension at a time (e.g., WARMTH). This will reduce the number of behaviors that must be observed to a more manageable level.

(Note that items 4, 5, 6, 8, and 27 are "one time only" behaviors. They are likely to occur only once during the interview either at the beginning or the end. Note also that all the AS-SERTIVENESS behaviors are negative. The more these behaviors are checked off, the less likely it is that the person you are observing is ASSERTIVE).

Questions for Discussion

- Which assessment method is easier to use: content analysis or rating scales?
- Which behaviors were most difficult to observe?
- What behaviors were you exhibiting that you were not aware of?
- What behaviors do you feel you need to use more in your interview?

3.   In What Type of Situation Should Interpersonal Skills Be Assessed?

It is possible to assess interpersonal skills by having students write what they think is a good response to a written patient-stimulus statement. This type of pencil and paper test shows whether the student has learned what a good response is, but it does not adequately test whether the student can make the response when responding to an actual person (Schwartz and Gottman, 1976). Knowing what to do and being able to do it are two different things. Similarly, interpersonal skill tests that focus on determining whether the student can identify good interpersonal skill responses (for example, the student is shown a typescript or videotape of health professional responses to a patient and must choose the best response) are similarly limited (Carkhuff, Collingwood, and Renz, 1969). Because of the limitations of paper and pencil tests and discrimination tests of interpersonal skills, we will instead focus on situations in which the ability of health professionals to actually demonstrate their interpersonal skills can be assessed.

There are three aspects to the type of situation in which interpersonal skills are assessed: who the interviewee is (patient, health professional student, or programmed patient), the realness of the problems discussed (actual versus role played), and how the interpersonal skills are observed (live, videotape, or audiotape).

Who the interviewee is. Generally speaking, it is more desirable to assess students' interpersonal skills in actual interviews with patients. Health professional students will ultimately have to demonstrate their interpersonal skills with patients and assessment of a student's interpersonal skills with actual patients is likely to be indicative of the way he will relate to other patients. The main disadvantage of assessing a student's interpersonal skills with patients is that if the student's interpersonal skills are not at a high level (3.0 or better), the patient may suffer. Being exposed to a health professional whose ACTIVE LISTENING, WARMTH, INITIATING, or ASSERTIVENESS skills are around the 1.0 to 1.5 level can be very aversive for patients. Another disadvantage of using patients is that the student must be assessed interviewing a large number of patients in order to determine the adequacy of the student's interpersonal skills in handling a range of problems (e.g., crying patients, aggressive patients, patients in pain, etc.). It is also difficult to compare scores for different students when each student has conducted an interview with different patients. A similar problem exists when comparing a student's scores before and after interpersonal skills training. Because the age, sex, and difficulty of patients vary, students' scores will vary as well. This makes score comparison difficult.

One advantage of using health professional students as "patients" is that they are readily accessible. Students taking a course in interpersonal skills can interview each other about real or role-played problems. The ease with which this type of assessment can be carried out makes it a useful formative evaluation of students' interpersonal skills. Formative evaluation is evaluation directed at giving the student ongoing feedback on how he is performing while he is learning a skill. Formative evaluation aids the student in determining the extent to which he is achieving his learning goals. Summative evaluation is conducted at the end of a training program and is used to test whether students have met key course objectives and to provide comparative information on students. Using students as "patients" is an excellent form of formative evaluation because of the accessibility of the students, the ease with which the "testing" can be carried out as part of regular classroom exercises in interpersonal skills, and the absence of risk to real patients. Using students as "patients," however, is an ineffective way of performing a summative evaluation because of the lack of standardization and because of problems in having students participate in a formal "test" of each other.

Some of these problems can be overcome using actors who role play patients with different problems. These "programmed patients" can be used to simulate a wide variety of common patient situations. This permits a more thorough testing of the health professional student's interpersonal skills across a range of situations. The use of programmed patients also standardizes somewhat the type of patient each student in an interpersonal skills course is tested on. This allows a more meaningful comparison between students' scores, since all students will have been exposed to "similar" patients. In addition, if a student's interpersonal skills are weak, there is no real threat to the "patient." The main disadvantage of using programmed patients is the cost involved in developing and maintaining a pool of "actors" who will role play a variety of patient situations.

The BEHAVIORAL TEST OF INTERPERSONAL SKILLS FOR HEALTH PROFESSIONALS (BTIS) is an interpersonal skills test that uses videotape to present patient situations to which the health professional student must respond, demonstrating his interpersonal skills (Gerrard, 1979). The BTIS is essentially a videotape presentation of programmed patients (and programmed health professionals).

The BTIS is intended to be used to assess the interpersonal/interviewing skills of any health professional or health professional student. The test consists of 30 common patient and health professional situations that have been role played by actors and recorded on videotape. An important feature of the BTIS is that it contains vignettes involving health professionals as well as patients. This permits an assessment of a student's "team skills" as well as his interpersonal skills for dealing with patients.

This test is called a behavioral test because it elicits a complete behavioral response from the student being tested. The student whose skills are being assessed sits in front of a TV monitor. As the TV plays back each of the recorded problem situations on the videotape (e.g., a crying patient, a patient in pain, or an aggressive health professional), the student must make a verbal response to the situation as though he were interacting with a real person. The patient or health professional "stimulus" is presented over a one-minute (approximate) interval. During the first 20–30 seconds, the patient or health professional speaks and responds nonverbally. During the last 30 seconds, the patient or health professional is silent but continues to respond (on TV) nonverbally (e.g., the patient may have a sad look on her face). During this same 30-second period, the student whose interpersonal skills are being assessed makes what he feels to be an appropriate response to the stimulus situation. The student's responses may be scored "live" or they can be videotaped and scored later. The BTIS can be scored for EMPATHY (ACTIVE LISTENING), WARMTH, INITIATING, and ASSERTIVENESS.

The BTIS was developed using the behavioral-analytic approach (Goldfried and D'Zurilla, 1969). The vignettes used in the BTIS were developed with the assistance of 68 experienced health professionals representing the main health professional disciplines. The 30 vignettes in the BTIS were distilled from an original list of 70 vignettes. The final set of vignettes represent a broad range of common interpersonal problems that health professionals have to deal with. The basic vignette design for the BTIS is shown in the table on the following page.

BASIC VIGNETTE DESIGN FOR BTIS

Category	Subcategory*	Number of Patient Vignettes	Number of Health Professional Vignettes
1. Aggression	Verbal Attack	2	2
	Unreasonable Request	2	2
2. Distress	Crying	2	—
	Pain	2	—
	Anxiety	2	2
	Anger	2	2
3. Positive Emotion	Happiness	2	2
	Affection	2	2
4. Performance Evaluation	Performance Evaluation	—	2
	TOTAL	16	14 = 30

* Each subcategory of vignette (e.g., Verbal Attack) has 2 vignettes representative of that subcategory, one role played by a male, the other by a female.

The BTIS takes approximately 30 minutes to take and the same length of time to rate (if ratings are done from videotape). The BTIS can be computer scored. A sample computer printout answer sheet with scores is shown on page 290. Ratings were made using the behaviorally anchored rating scales for EMPATHY (ACTIVE LISTENING), WARMTH, INITIATING, and ASSERTIVENESS. Numbers in parentheses refer to specific vignettes in the BTIS. The symbol P refers to patient vignettes; HP refers to health professional vignettes. The number 9.9 is used to indicate vignettes that are not scored for a particular interpersonal skill. The answer sheet shows that Ann obtained overall mean scores of 2.50 for EMPATHY; 2.86 for WARMTH, 3.04 for INITIATING, and 3.13 for ASSERTIVENESS. Although Ann has demonstrated minimum competence on INITIATING and ASSERTIVENESS, she scored low on WARMTH and on EMPATHY.

The advantage of the BTIS over other methods of assessing interpersonal skills is that it is a *standardized* measure of actual (although role played) behavior in response to a *wide variety* of

SCORE SHEET FOR BEHAVIORAL TEST OF
INTERPERSONAL SKILLS FOR HEALTH PROFESSIONALS

August 7, 1979   Subject: ANN   Rated by: JIM

Scene	Empathy	Warmth	Initiating	Assertiveness
3	2.0	2.0	3.5	9.9
4	3.0	3.0	3.5	3.0
5	3.0	3.0	9.9	9.9
6	9.9	3.0	3.5	9.9
7	2.5	2.5	2.5	3.0
8	2.5	3.0	3.0	3.0
9	1.5	3.0	3.0	9.9
10	2.0	2.0	3.0	9.9
11	9.9	3.0	9.9	9.9
12	2.5	3.0	3.0	9.9
13	2.5	3.0	2.5	9.9
14	3.0	3.0	9.9	9.9
15	2.5	3.0	3.5	9.9
16	3.0	3.0	9.9	9.9
17	1.5	3.0	3.0	9.9
18	3.0	3.0	3.0	3.0
19	2.5	3.0	9.9	9.9
20	2.5	2.5	2.5	3.5
21	2.5	3.0	3.0	9.9
22	9.9	3.0	9.9	9.9
23	2.0	2.5	3.0	9.9
24	3.5	3.0	2.5	9.9
25	9.9	3.0	3.0	9.9
26	2.5	2.0	3.0	3.0
27	9.9	3.0	9.9	9.9
28	2.5	3.0	3.5	9.9
29	9.9	3.0	9.9	9.9
30	2.5	2.5	3.0	3.0
31	3.0	3.0	3.0	9.9
32	2.5	3.0	3.0	3.5

interpersonal problems commonly faced by health professionals. The standardized nature of the BTIS makes it particularly useful for summative assessment, for comparing the interpersonal skills of different students, for comparing the interpersonal skills of the same student before and after training, for admissions screening, and for research on interpersonal skills.

ANSWER SHEET FOR BTIS

Main Category	Sub-Category	Empathy P	HP	T	Warmth P	HP	T	Initiating P	HP	T	Assertiveness P	HP	T
Aggression	Verbal Attack P(4,7), HP(18,26)	2.75	2.75	2.75	2.75	2.50	2.63	3.00	3.00	3.00	3.00	3.00	3.00
	Unreasonable Request P(30,32), HP(8,20)	2.50	2.50	2.50	2.75	2.75	2.75	3.00	2.75	2.88	3.25	3.25	3.25
	Mean Aggression			2.63			2.69			2.94			3.13
Distress	Crying P(28,31)	2.75		2.75	3.00		3.00	3.25		3.25			
	Pain P(17,13)	2.00		2.00	3.00		3.00	2.75		2.75			
	Anxiety P(9,12) HP(15,23)	2.00	2.25	2.13	3.00	2.75	2.88	3.00	3.25	3.13			
	Anger P(3,24) HP(10,21)	2.75	2.25	2.50	2.50	2.50	2.50	3.00	3.00	3.00			
	Mean Distress			2.34			2.84			3.03			
Positive Emotion	Happiness P(5,19) HP(14,16)	2.75	3.00	2.88	3.00	3.00	3.00						
	Affection P(27,29) HP(11,22)				3.00	3.00	3.00						
	Mean			2.88			3.00						
Performance Evaluation HP(6,25)						3.00	3.00		3.25	3.25			
	Overall Mean	2.50	2.55	2.50	2.88	2.79	2.86	3.00	3.05	3.04	3.13	3.13	3.13

The realness of the problems discussed. When assessing interpersonal skills, it is important that the interview situation be as real as possible. The closer the assessment situation is to the actual interview conditions in which the health professional student will be working, the more it will be possible to generalize the results of the assessment. Generally speaking, it is preferable to assess students' interpersonal skills using patients or students who talk about real problems. "Realness," however, is largely in the mind of the beholder. If a programmed patient can give a convincing performance as (say) a depressed patient, then that situation will be real for the student who is being assessed.

How the interpersonal skills are observed. The person who is assessing a student's interpersonal skills can "observe" the student in three main ways. He can view the actual interview through a one-way mirror, or observe the student directly in the actual room where the interview is being conducted. Second, he can view and score a videotape of the student's interview. And third, he can listen to and score an audiotape of the student's interview. Of these three methods, listening to an audiotape is the least satisfactory because the observer cannot see the body language of the interviewer. This reduces the reliability with which WARMTH and ASSERTIVENESS can be scored because these two interpersonal skills are largely communicated through the health professional's body language. Videotape has the advantage that the observer can replay sections of the interview to check his scoring. The videotape can also be used to give explicit feedback to the student on those portions of the interview in which he did well or poorly. Having an observer sit in the actual interviewing room has the disadvantage of making both the student and the patient more anxious. This is not as critical a problem, however, when a formative assessment is made in the classroom using students as subjects and as observers. Observing a student through a one-way mirror has the advantage of minimizing the reactive effects of having an observer physically present in the interview room. Some patients may be a little nervous at first about the one-way mirror, but giving them the explanation that use of the one-way mirror is normal clinic procedure and an aid to helping the health professional student improve his skill will have a calming effect.

The relative merits of using patients, students, programmed patients, or the BEHAVIORAL TEST OF INTERPERSONAL SKILLS FOR HEALTH PROFESSIONALS (BTIS) to assess students' interpersonal skills are shown in the table that follows.

	Assessment Characteristics	*Stimulus Used To Elicit Students' Interpersonal Skills*			
		Patients	Students	Programmed Patients	BTIS
1.	Interviews can be videotaped	++	++	++	++
2.	Low risk for patients	-	++	++	++
3.	Useful for formative evaluation	+	++	+	-
4.	Useful for summative evaluation	+	-	++	++
5.	Standardized	-	-	+	++
6.	Wide range of problems presented	-	+	+	++
7.	Interviewer can interact with interviewee	+	+	+	-
8.	Feasibility (low cost, ease of implementation)	+	++	-	+

Legend: ++ = Assessment characteristic is present to a high degree.
         +   = Assessment characteristic is present to a moderate degree.
         -   = Assessment characteristic is present to a low degree.

One way a comprehensive assessment of health professional students' interpersonal skills could be made during different phases of training is shown below.

		Phase of Interpersonal Skills Training		
		Pretest	During Training	Post-Test
1.	Stimulus used to elicit students' interpersonal skills.	BTIS or Programmed Patients	Students (Peers)	BTIS or Programmed Patients, Real Patients.
2.	Assessment method	Rating Scales Content Analysis	Written Feedback Rating Scales Content Analysis	Rating Scales Content Analysis Patient Feedback Form

In this assessment design, the same pretest and post-test measure is used (BTIS or Programmed Patients) for summative evaluation. Students are used as "patients" to provide formative evaluation during training. Patients are also used for summative post-test assessment as a "real life" check and to ensure actual transfer of skills to clinic situations.

4. Who Should Assess Interpersonal Skills?

A student's interpersonal skills may be assessed by the student himself, his fellow students, his supervisor (or another faculty member), or the "patient." Ideally all four rating sources will be involved in the assessment of any one student. The value of having a student rate his own performance in an interview is that it helps him to learn to make a more accurate self-assessment through comparing his self-ratings with those of others. The value of having students rate each other is that it helps them to learn to discriminate good interpersonal skills. The student's supervisor (instructor, faculty member) should rate his student because his greater experience and skill, plus his individual knowledge of the particular student, will help him (hopefully) to make a more objective rating. The advantage of having the "patient" rate the student's interpersonal skills is that it serves to confirm the extent to which the students interpersonal skills actually made an impact on the patient. Health professionals rarely get this type of valuable patient feedback. For making a formative evaluation of a student's interpersonal skills, assessment by the student himself and by his fellow students is acceptable. Self- and peer ratings, however, are not desirable when making a summative evaluation of students' interpersonal skills. When making a summative evaluation, supervisor (or faculty) ratings should be used. If instructors wish to eliminate from the assessment of their students possible bias caused by knowing the student, they can rate each others' students.

Exercise 53:   Patient Feedback on Interpersonal Skills

Purpose: To develop skills in obtaining patient feedback on your interpersonal skills.

Instructions: 1. Xerox several copies of the Patient Feedback Form and Results Sheet.

2. Arrange with the secretary of the clinic in which you are interviewing patients to ask each of your patients to complete the Patient Feedback Form on you following his interview with you.

3. Score your Patient Feedback Forms using the Results Sheet provided.

4. Share your patient feedback with another student (or your supervisor).

Questions for Discussion

•   How do your patient feedback scores correlate with ratings of your interpersonal skills made by yourself, your supervisor, or your peers?

•   What do your patients see as your weakest interpersonal skills? Strongest interpersonal skills?

PATIENT FEEDBACK FORM

_____ , the student who you just had your interview with, is a learner in our clinic and is very interested in learning what patients think and feel about how he/she conducts his/her interview. Would you please take a moment and rate this student on how well the interview with you went. Do this by placing a check mark (✓) in the appropriate column to the right to indicate how much you agree or disagree with each statement listed below. Be sure to rate each statement.

Use the opposite side of this page to write down any comments you wish to make about your interview.

	6 Strongly Agree	5 Moderately Agree	4 Slightly Agree	3 Slightly Disagree	2 Moderately Disagree	1 Strongly Disagree
1. The student was friendly.						
2. I would be willing to see this student again.						
3. The student asked me if I had any questions.						
4. The student was interested in what I had to say.						
5. The student understood my feelings.						
6. The student was confident.						
7. The student answered my questions.						
8. The student seemed relaxed.						
9. The student knows what to do to help me.						
10. The student did a good job.						
11. I am satisfied with the way the interview went.						
12. The student understood my worries.						
13. I believe the treatment I received today will help me.						
14. I would recommend this student to my friends.						

RESULTS SHEET FOR PATIENT FEEDBACK FORM

Instructions: For items 1 to 14 score all Strongly Agree responses as 6, all Moderately Agree responses as 5, ... all Strongly Disagree responses as 1. Total up your scores as shown below.

Score

ACTIVE LISTENING
(Add 5 + 12)   14

WARMTH
(Add 1 + 4)   14

RESPECT
(Add 3 + 7)   14

INITIATING
(Add 9 + 10)   14

ASSERTIVENESS
(Add 6 + 8)   14

PATIENT SATISFACTION
(Add 2, 11, 13, 14)   28

5. How Is the Reliability of the Assessment Method To be Determined?

RELIABILITY is one of the most important concepts in measurement. RELIABILITY refers to how consistent a measuring instrument is.

Example

Joan and Luis, two health professional instructors, decide to rate the INITIATING skills of five of their students. Joan and Luis watch a videotape made by each student and assign a score using the behaviorally anchored rating for INITIATING. The results of the ratings are shown below.

Rating made by:

Student	Joan	Luis	
1	3.5	3.5	
2	2.5	2.5	
3	4.0	4.0	
4	3.0	3.0	
5	1.5	1.0	(r = .99)

As can be seen, Joan's and Luis' ratings are almost exactly the same. Their ratings are consistent and therefore reliable.

Measuring instruments that are not reliable are inconsistent. An inconsistent measuring instrument is like a rubber ruler that changes its length each time you use it to measure something. The scores obtained from an unreliable measuring instrument have no clear meaning. We cannot put our confidence in them.

Example

Martin and Sheila, two health professionals who teach in the same program as Joan and Luis, have also been teaching a course in interpersonal skills to a group of five students. Martin and Sheila rate their students on INITIATING skills and obtain the following scores.

Rating made by:

Student	Martin	Sheila	
6	1.0	3.0	
7	3.5	1.5	
8	4.0	2.0	
9	2.0	4.0	
10	1.5	2.5	(r = -.64)

There is no consistency between Martin's ratings and Sheila's ratings. Students rated by Martin as high on INITIATING are rated by Sheila as low on INITIATING. Martin and Sheila are unable to agree on what is good and what is poor INITIATING. Their ratings are unreliable and therefore useless for assessment purposes.

There are two main types of reliability: INTER-RATER RE-
LIABILITY and INTRA-RATER RELIABILITY. Inter-rater reliability refers to the extent of agreement between raters (this is
illustrated in the two examples above). Intra-rater reliability refers
to the consistency with which the same rater scores the same
student videotape (for example) on two different occasions.

Example

Joan decides to determine her intra-rater reliability. One
week after rating the five students' videotapes with Luis,
Joan views and scores the same five videotapes. Her
scores are shown below:

Joan's ratings:

Student	First time	Second time	
1	3.5	3.5	
2	2.5	2.5	
3	4.0	4.0	
4	3.0	3.5	
5	1.5	1.0	$(r = .86)$

Joan's ratings on the two different occasions are virtually identical. Her ratings are consistent; she has high
intra-rater reliability.

Example

Martin waits one week and then rescores his tapes in
order to determine his intra-rater reliability. His scores
are:

Martin's ratings:

Student	First time	Second time	
6	1.0	3.0	
7	3.5	2.0	
8	4.0	2.5	
9	2.0	3.5	
10	1.5	2.5	$(r = -.56)$

There is no consistency between Martin's ratings
across time. His intra-rater reliability is very low. This
means that ratings of INITIATING given by Martin are

inaccurate and meaningless as feedback for students (or faculty).

There are several ways of calculating reliability. One of the most popular methods is the Pearson product-moment correlation coefficient, which is symbolized by the letter r. The Pearson product-moment correlation coefficient varies from +1.00 to –1.00. A score of + 1.00 indicates a strong positive relationship between the scores given by two raters to the same students. A "positive relationship" means that when rater A scores a student high, rater B will also tend to score that same student high. When rater A scores a student low, rater B also tends to score that student low. A score of – 1.00 indicates a strong negative relationship between two sets of scores. A "negative relationship" means that when rater A scores a student high, rater B will tend to score that same student low, and vice versa. The formula for calculating the Pearson product-moment correlation coefficient can be found in almost any introductory textbook on statistics. For each example shown in this section, a Pearson r is shown in brackets.

A reliability coefficient of .80 is generally accepted as the minimum acceptable level for rating students' interpersonal skills. If your reliability is below .80, this means your ratings are likely to be inaccurate. Ratings for a summative evaluation of students should not be used unless the raters have first demonstrated both inter-rater and intra-rater reliabilities of .80 or above.

One disadvantage in using Pearson r to compute your reliability is that r merely shows the strength of the relationship between two sets of scores. For example, both sets of scores shown below have the same Pearson r.

Students	Rater A	Rater B	
1	4.0	4.0	
2	3.0	3.0	
3	3.5	3.5	
4	2.5	2.5	
5	3.5	3.5	$(r = 1.00)$

Students	Rater C	Rater D	
1	4.0	3.0	
2	3.0	2.0	
3	3.5	2.5	
4	2.5	1.5	
5	3.5	2.5	$(r = 1.00)$

The reliability coefficient for raters A and B is 1.00, and there is no difference between the scores for any one student. The reliability coefficient for raters C and D is also 1.00 (when C's ratings are high, so are D's; when C's ratings are low, so are D's), but there is a difference of 1.0 between C and D for each student rated. This means that rater D is consistently rating the students lower than C. For this reason, a statistical test called the *t-test* should be used to check out whether the scores of two raters differ. That is, every time you calculate a Pearson *r* for two sets of ratings, you should also make a *t-test* for those same ratings.

A minimal procedure for determining the reliability with which you are able to use a rating scale is:

Step 1:   View and rate (e.g., using a behaviorally anchored rating scale) at least 15 videotape segments representing a range of good and of poor interpersonal skills as demonstrated by several students (the greater the number of different students you can use for your reliability check, the better).

Step 2:   Have an experienced health professional (ideally one who teaches interpersonal skills) view and rate the same 15 videotape segments using the same rating scale.

Step 3:   Compute a Pearson product-moment correlation and a *t-test* for the two sets of scores. If your Pearson *r* is at least .80 and the *t-test* shows that there is no significant difference between the scores, you have attained adequate inter-rater reliability. If the Pearson *r* is less than .80, or the *t-test* shows that your scores are significantly different, you should meet with the other rater, practice rating a new sample of videotapes together until you reach satisfactory agreement in your ratings, and then retest your reliability (repeat steps 1 and 2) on a new set of 15 videotapes. This retraining and retesting procedure must be repeated until satisfactory reliability is reached.

Step 4:   After one week, view and rerate the 15 videotapes you rated in STEP 1. Calculate your intra-rater reliability (do STEP 3). If the Pearson *r* is below

.80 or the *t-test* indicates that your scores differ, further retraining and retesting will be necessary.

For a more detailed review of methodological issues in determining reliability (especially rater bias and how to avoid it) see Kent and Foster (1977).

An alternative way to calculate rater reliability is to use a statistic called Kappa (Cohen, 1960). This is a very stringent reliability coefficient because it includes a correction for chance agreement between raters.

6. Is the Assessment Method Valid?

The term *validity* refers to whether an assessment method measures what it is supposed to measure. For example, the length of time it takes your heart rate to return to normal following exercise is a more valid indicator of the healthy state of your heart than is a measurement of your height (which would have little validity as a measure of the health status of your heart). In the 1840's phrenology—the art of diagnosing personality by feeling the bumps and hollows on a person's head—was a widely used technique. However, as a method of assessing personality it had no validity. It simply didn't measure what it was supposed to.

An assessment method may be reliable but still lack validity. For example, a ruler can be used to accurately measure a patient's height because it is a reliable instrument for measuring height. But it cannot be used to assess a patient's overall health status because it lacks validity for measuring health status. An assessment method that is reliable but lacks validity is like a person who always tells the same lie but does so with great consistency.

An understanding of the concept of validity is important when choosing an assessment method for measuring interpersonal skills. If the assessment method chosen lacks validity, the scores obtained from it will have no practical meaning. In everyday speech the phrase, "Is it valid?" is taken to mean, "Is it true?" The term *validity*, as applied to methods of assessing interpersonal skills, has a similar concern with the "truthfulness" of the assessment method. In this sense, an assessment method that lacks validity is one that "lies" to us. The problem is: How can we determine whether an assessment method is telling the "truth"? The answer is: We try to collect as much evidence as we can for the validity ("truthfulness") of the assessment method we are using.

There are three main types of validity for which an assessment method can be examined:

CONTENT VALIDITY

CRITERION-RELATED VALIDITY

CONSTRUCT VALIDITY

CONTENT VALIDITY refers to the extent to which the student skills assessed in a particular test are representative of the actual skills the student will have to demonstrate in "real life."

Example of a test with Poor CONTENT VALIDITY: An IQ test that assesses *only* skills in arithmetic. This test would lack CONTENT VALIDITY because it assesses only *one* aspect of intelligence. (However, as a test of arithmetical reasoning it might have high CONTENT VALIDITY.)

Example of a test with Excellent CONTENT VALIDITY: The Wechsler Adult Intelligence Scale (WAIS) assesses a wide range of different aspects of intelligence. It consists of the following eleven sub-tests:

Verbal Sub-tests

1. General Information	3. Arithmetical Reasoning
2. General Comprehension	4. Similarities
	5. Digit Span
	6. Vocabulary

Performance Sub-tests

7. Digit Symbol	10. Picture Arrangement
8. Picture Completion	11. Object Assembly
9. Block Design	

There are two aspects of CONTENT VALIDITY that relate to the assessment of interpersonal skills. First, there is the CONTENT VALIDITY of the interpersonal skills assessment method with respect to the types of interpersonal problems on which the student is assessed. That is, is the student assessed on his skill in handling only one or two common interpersonal problems (e.g., the patient in pain, the depressed patient)? Or is the student assessed on a more complete range of interpersonal problems typical of those he will encounter as a practicing health professional (e.g., patients who are in pain, depressed, angry, manipulative, happy, affectionate, aggressive, or anxious; other health professionals who are angry, aggressive, critical, manipulative, happy, or affectionate)? Second, there is the CONTENT VALIDITY of the rating scale or content analysis system that is used to assess the student's responses to the problem situations with which he is presented. That is, is the student assessed on only one interpersonal skill (e.g., INITIATING), or is the student assessed on a wide range of critical interpersonal skills (e.g., ACTIVE LISTENING, WARMTH, INITIATING, and ASSERTIVENESS)?

In summary, the CONTENT VALIDITY of an interpersonal skills "test" refers to:

1. The *problem situations* used to elicit the student's interpersonal skills, and
2. The specific *interpersonal skills* that are assessed (usually by a rating scale or a content analysis system).

If an interpersonal skills assessment method has high CONTENT VALIDITY, it will sample a wide range of common interpersonal *problem situations* and a wide range of *interpersonal skills* that are relevant to practicing health professionals.

CRITERION-RELATED VALIDITY refers to the extent to which an individual's scores on a test correlate witth the individual's scores on a criterion that is a direct and independent measure of what the test was designed to measure.

There are two types of CRITERION-RELATED VALIDITY: CONCURRENT VALIDITY and PREDICTIVE VALIDITY. CONCURRENT VALIDITY refers to the extent to which an individual's scores on a test corresponds to the individual's *current* scores on an independent "criterion" measure. The criterion is the standard against which the "truthfulness" of the test is compared. For example, a health professional might determine the CONCURRENT VALIDITY of a test of a patient's health status (e.g., a questionnaire completed by patients) by correlating patients' scores on the new test with *ratings* assigned by a group of experienced health professionals for each patient's degree of well-being. The judges' ratings of patients' health status is the criterion against which the new test is compared. If the "new" test correlates well with the expert ratings, this suggests that the new test has CONCURRENT VALIDITY. It should be noted that validity coefficients are usually in the .30–.40 range. This is because the criterion test usually only partly measures the attribute in question. Indeed, this is one of the reasons for constructing a new test—to measure an attribute more accurately than "old" tests permit.

PREDICTIVE VALIDITY refers to the ability of a test to predict the performance of an individual on a criterion measure (e.g., a test) taken after a time interval. For example, if students who have good high school grades also obtain good grades in the first year of a health professional program, this suggests that high school grades have PREDICTIVE VALIDITY. They predict a student's future performance. With respect to this subject, Hoyt (1965) analyzed 46 studies and concluded that college grades bore little or no relationship to any measures of adult accomplishment. Ericksen and Bluestone (1960) report that studies relating undergraduate grades to first-year grades in graduate and professional schools have produced correlations of about .30. Ericksen and Bluestone state:

> Predictions of grades beyond the first graduate year are even lower, and predictions of grades in clinically oriented programs are little better than chance. (Ericksen and Bluestone, 1971, p. 125).

This suggests that undergraduate grades have low predictive validity for success in graduate programs (an interesting fact, considering the number of health professional programs that rely solely on undergraduate grades for admitting students).

CONSTRUCT VALIDITY is the most complex type of validity. The CONSTRUCT VALIDITY of a test is the extent to which the test measures a particular theoretical construct. A construct is an abstract variable (e.g., intelligence) that is measured through some manifestation of behavior (e.g., performance on a vocabulary or arithmetic test). The interpersonal skill WARMTH, for example, is a construct (idea) used to describe a variety of behaviors that seem to go together (e.g., smiling, warm voice tone, friendly facial expression, paying attention to what the other person is saying, saying considerate things to the other person, etc.).

A test has CONSTRUCT VALIDITY if it behaves in ways we logically expect it to behave in relation to other measures (tests).

There are two main types of CONSTRUCT VALIDITY: CONVERGENT VALIDITY and DISCRIMINANT VALIDITY. A test has CONVERGENT VALIDITY if it correlates highly with variables with which it should theoretically and logically correlate. A test has DISCRIMINANT VALIDITY if it doesn't correlate highly with variables with which it should theoretically and logically differ. For example, evidence for the CONVERGENT VALIDITY of IQ tests comes from their moderate to high correlation with grades. Evidence for the DISCRIMINANT VALIDITY of IQ tests comes from their non-significant correlation with most personality tests. In both instances, IQ scores correlate with other variables in predicted directions. This is evidence of CONSTRUCT VALIDITY.

A test has CONVERGENT VALIDITY if it distinguishes in an expected way between two groups known to be different. For example, the BEHAVIORAL TEST OF INTERPERSONAL SKILLS (BTIS) was administered to the 1979 class of 12 Master of Health Science students at McMaster University and to an equal number of randomly selected first-year nurses at McMaster University. The mean number of BTIS vignettes on which the Master of Health Science students made FEELING REFLECTION responses was 11.8 (out of a possible 24 vignettes), compared to a mean score of 6.8 obtained by the first-year nurses. It is reasonable to expect that the Master of Health Science students would perform better and, in fact, they did. (The difference was statistically significant at the .004 level, for a t-test.) This is an example of CONVERGENT VALIDITY by the known groups method.

A second type of CONVERGENT VALIDITY comes from examining the effect of experimental variables on test scores. We would expect health professional students who have taken an intensive course in interpersonal skills to receive higher scores on an interpersonal skills test than those students who have not taken the course (especially when the students have been randomly assigned to both "treatment" and "control" groups). When an interpersonal skills test discriminates between students who have been specifically taught interpersonal skills and those who have not, this suggests that the test has CONSTRUCT VALIDITY. We expect the test to discriminate, and it does.

Example

In 1979, 30 first-year nurses at McMaster University were randomly assigned to 4 treatment groups (of 7 students each) and 1 control group (containing 10 students). The 4 treatment groups received a 6 week (12 hour) intensive course in interpersonal skills, with particular emphasis on the skill of ACTIVE LISTENING. Students in the control group did not receive the course. The following scores were obtained on the BTIS for the content analysis category REFLECTS FEELINGS. These scores represent the number of vignettes—out of a possible 24—for which students successfully reflected the feelings of the "patient" or "health professional" in the vignette.

	Group 1	Group 2	Group 3	Group 4	Control Group
	11	13	22	22	5
	17	16	7	20	7
	15	11	17	21	8
	21	18	17	18	7
	16	18	13	20	13
	16	14	12	7	6
	16	11	19	20	7
					7
					7
					4
Total	112	101	107	128	71
x̄	16.0	14.4	15.3	18.3	7.1

The lowest scoring treatment group performed twice as well as the control group. The differences between the treatment groups and the control group are statistically significant. This suggests further evidence for the CONSTRUCT VALIDITY of the BTIS for the interpersonal skill REFLECTS FEELINGS.

The more evidence we can accumulate that demonstrates the CONVERGENT and DISCRIMINANT VALIDITY of a test, the more assured we can be that the test has CONSTRUCT VALIDITY (that the construct we want to measure is in fact being measured).

The different types of validity and examples of the kinds of evidence used to indicate the presence of each type of validity are summarized below.

Type of Validity	Examples of Evidence of Validity for an Interpersonal Skills "Test"
1. CONTENT	Judge's ratings of the relevancy of the interpersonal *problem situations* assessed.
	Judge's ratings of the relevancy of the *interpersonal skills* assessed.

Theoretical and experimental evidence that provides a rationale for the inclusion of specific interpersonal problem situations and interpersonal skills.

2. CRITERION-RELATED
    (a) CONCURRENT

Judge's ratings of students' interpersonal skills demonstrated in actual patient interviews (which are then correlated with scores from the interpersonal skills "test"), when both the ratings and the interpersonal skills "test" are made during the same two-week period.

    (b) PREDICTIVE

Judge's ratings of students' interpersonal skills demonstrated in actual patient interviews (which are correlated with scores from the interpersonal skills "test" which was administered as an admissions screening test one year earlier).

3. CONSTRUCT
    (a) CONVERGENT

Scores obtained on the interpersonal skills test by first year students are compared with scores obtained by graduate students.

Scores obtained on the interpersonal skills test by students who have completed an interpersonal skills course are compared with the scores obtained by a control group of students who have not received the interpersonal skills course.

There is a moderate positive correlation between scores obtained by students on the interpersonal skills test and scores obtained by the same students on another test of interpersonal skills.

    (b) DISCRIMINANT

There is a non-significant correlation between scores obtained by students on the interpersonal skills test and scores obtained by the same students on a test that has no logical or theoretical connection with interpersonal skills (e.g., a test of physical strength).

SUMMARY

Health professionals assess interpersonal skills for several reasons: to evaluate their own interpersonal skills so that they can keep their skills "sharp," to perform formative and summative evaluations of students, to evaluate the quality of programs used to teach interpersonal skills, to screen applicants for health professional programs, and to conduct research on the impact of health professionals' interpersonal skills on patients. The six key issues in the assessment of interpersonal skills are: what interpersonal skills should be assessed, how should interpersonal skills be assessed, in what type of situation should interpersonal skills be assessed, who should do the assessing, how should reliability of the assessment method be determined, and is the assessment method valid. Four key interpersonal skills that health professionals should assess are: ACTIVE LISTENING (EMPATHY), WARMTH, ASSERTIVENESS, and INITIATING. The three main methods of assessing these interpersonal skills are written feedback, rating scales, and content analysis. The BEHAVIORAL TEST OF INTERPERSONAL SKILLS FOR HEALTH PROFESSIONALS is a standardized test that can be used to determine whether health professional students have learned specific interpersonal skills. Irregardless of whether real patients, students, or programmed patients are used as the stimulus to elicit students' interpersonal skills, rater reliability should always be determined if a summative evaluation is being made.

References

References for Chapter 1

Aluise, J. "Human relations training for family practice residents: a four year retrospective review." *The Journal of Family Practice* (1977) 4:881–88.

Balint, M. "The family doctor and patients' secrets." *Psychiatry in Medicine* (1971) 2:98–107.

Baer, E.; Davitz, L.; and Lieb, R. "Inferences of physical pain and psychological distress: 1. in relation to verbal and nonverbal patient communication." *Nursing Research* (1970) 19:388–92.

Becker, M.; Drachman, R.; and Kirscht, J. "Motivations as predictors of health behavior." *Health Services Reports* (1972) 87:852–62.

———. "Predicting mothers' compliance with pediatric medical regimens." *The Journal of Pediatrics* (1972) 81: 843-54.

Ben-Sira, Z. "The functions of the professional's affective behavior in client satisfaction: a revised approach to social interaction theory." *Journal of Health and Social Behavior* (1976) 17:3–11.

Bloom, M. "Interviewing the ill aged." *Gerontologist* (1971) 11:292–99.

Brown, R.; Wilkins, M.; Buxton, W.; and Abse, D. "Psychological factors in the etiology of lung cancer." *Virginia Medical Monthly* (1975) 102(11):935–39.

Carstairs, V. *Channels of Communication.* Edinburgh: Scottish Home and Health Department, 1970.

Cartwright, A. *Human Relations and Hospital Care.* London: Routledge & Kegan Paul, 1964.

Cassileth, B. "Surviving: staff adaptations to stress on a cancer ward." Unpublished doctoral dissertation, University of Pennsylvania, 1978.

Cline, D. and Garrard, J. "A medical interviewing course: objectives, techniques and assessment." *American Journal of Psychiatry* (1973) 130:85.

Coburn, D. and Jovaisas, A. "Perceived sources of stress among first-year medical students." *Journal of Medical Education* (1975) 59:589–95.

Conine, T. "Listening in the helping relationship." *Physical Therapy* February 19, 1976, 56:159-62.

Davidson, R. "Disturbed behavior in the older patient." *Practitioner* (1975) 215:600-605.

Davitz, L. "Identification of stressful situations in a Nigerian school of nursing." *Nursing Research* (1972) 21:352-57.

Duff, R. and Hollingshead, A. *Sickness and Society*. New York: Harper & Row, 1968.

Dye, M. "Clarifying patients' communications." *The American Journal of Nursing* (1963) 63:56-59.

Eldred, S. "Improving nurse-patient communication." *The American Journal of Nursing* (1960) 60:1600-1602.

Elstein, A.; Kagan, N.; and Shulman, L. "Methods and theory in the study of medical inquiry." *Journal of Medical Education* (1972) 47:85.

Fairchild, D. "Student nurses' avoidance of dying patients: death anxiety versus statement emotionality." Unpublished doctoral dissertation, University of Miami, 1977.

Feifel, H. "Physicians consider death." In *Proceedings, 75th Annual Convention*, American Psychological Association. Washington, D.C.: American Psychological Association, 1967.

Forster, B. and Forster, F. "Nursing students' reaction to the crying patient." *Nursing Research* (1971) 20:265-68.

Forsyth, G. "Exploration of empathy in nurse-client interaction." Unpublished doctoral dissertation, Texas Women's University, 1977.

Froelich, R. "A course in medical interviewing." *Journal of Medical Education* (1969) 44:1165-69.

Gerrard, B. "Interpersonal skills for health professionals: a review of the literature." Unpublished manuscript, Department of Medicine, McMaster University, 1978.

Goldin, P. and Russell, B. "Therapeutic communication." *The American Journal of Nursing* (1969) 69:1928-30.

Graffam, S. "Nurse response to the patient in distress—development of an instrument." *Nursing Research* (1970) 19:331-36.

Hampe, S. "Needs of the grieving spouse in a hospital setting." *Nursing Research* (1975) 24:113-20.

Heffner, W. "Medical staff counselors aid nursing students." *Hospital Topics* (1967) 45:44-46.

Helfer, R.; Black, M.; and Helfer, M.   "Pediatric interviewing skills taught by non-physicians." *American Journal of Diseases of Children* (1975) 129:1053-57.

Helfer, R.   "An objective comparison of the pediatric interviewing skills of freshman and senior medical students." *Pediatrics* (1970) 45:623-27.

Hetherington, R.; Ley, P.; Spelman, M.; and Jones, C.   "Research into the psychological effects of physical illness: interim report." Unpublished manuscript. Report to Nuffield Provincial Hospitals Trust, 1963.

Heymann, D.   "Discussions meet needs of dying patients." *Hospitals* (1974) 48(14):57-62.

Himmelhock, J.; Davies, R.; Tucker, G.; and Alderman, D.   "Butting heads: patients who refuse necessary procedures." *Psychiatry in Medicine* (1970) 1:241-49.

Hoekelman, R.   "Nurse-physician relationships." *American Journal of Nursing* (1975) 75:1150-52.

Houghton, H.   "Problems in hospital communication." In G. McLachlan (Ed.), *Problems and progress in medical care.* London: Oxford University Press, 1968.

Hugh Jones, P.; Tanser, A.; and Whitby, C.   "Patients' view of admission to a London teaching hospital." *British Medical Journal* (1964) 2:660-64.

Irwin, B. and Meier, J.   "Supportive measures for relatives of the fatally ill." *Comm. Nursing Research* (December 1973) 6119-28.

Jackson, J.   "Communication is important." *The American Journal of Nursing* (1959) 39:90-93.

Jason, H.; Kagan, N.; Werner, A.; Elstein, A.; and Thomas, J.   "New approaches to teaching basic interview skills to medical students." *American Journal of Psychology* (1970) 127:1404-07.

Jourard, S.   "Bedside manner." *American Journal of Nursing* (1960) 60:63-66.

Kales, J. and Kales, A.   "Managing the individual and family in crisis." *American Family Physician* (1975) 12:109-15.

Katz, S.   "The patients doctors hate to treat." *The Toronto Star* October 21, 1978, C4.

Kelly, N. and Menolascino, F.   "Physicians' awareness and attitudes towards the retarded." *Mental Retardation* (1975) 13(6):10-13.

Kiely, W. "Psychotherapy for the family physician." *American Family Physician* (1971) 3:87-91.

Kimball, C. "Interviewing, diagnosis and therapy." *Postgraduate Medicine* (1970) 47:88-93.

———. "Techniques of interviewing: setting up an interviewing course." *Psychiatry in Medicine* (1970) 1:167-70.

Kincey, J.; Bradshaw, P.; and Ley, P. "Patients' satisfaction and reported acceptance of advice in general practice." *Journal of the Royal College of General Practitioners* (1975) 25:558-66.

Klein, R. "The patient's feelings." *American Family Physician* (1974) 10:198-200.

Knowles, L. "How can we reassure patients?" *American Journal of Nursing* (1959) 59:832-35.

Korsch, B. and Negrete, V. "Doctor-patient communication." *Scientific American* (1972) 227:66-74.

Kowalewski, E. "Viewpoint: counseling often is vital tool in medical therapy." *Geriatrics* (1972) 27:32-40.

Krebs, R. "Disrespect—A study in hospital relationships." *Hospitals and Health Services Administration* (1976) 21:67-72.

Kubler-Ross, E. "The care of the dying—whose job is it?" *Psychiatry in Medicine* (1970) 47:88-93.

Lamonica, E.; Carew, D.; Winder, A.; Haase, A.; and Blanchard, K. "Empathy training as the major thrust of a staff development program." *Nursing Research* (1976) 25:447-51.

Lester, D.; Getty, C.; and Kneisl, C. "Attitudes of nursing students and nursing faculty toward death." *Nursing Research* (1974) 23:50-53.

Ley, P. and Spelman, M. *Communicating with the Patient.* St. Louis: Warren H. Green, 1967.

Liptak, G.; Hulka, B.; and Cassel, J. "Effectiveness of physician-mother interactions during infancy." *The Journal of Pediatrics* (1977) 60:186-92.

Loch, W. "The doctor-patient relationship in general practice: implications for diagnosis and treatment." *Pschiatry in Medicine* (1972) 3:365-70.

Lorber, J. "Good patients and problem patients: conformity and deviance in a general hospital." *Journal of Health and Social Behavior* (1975) 213-25.

Ludy, J.; Gagnon, J.; and Caiola, S. "The patient-pharmacist interaction in two ambulatory settings: its relationship to patient satisfaction and drug misuse." *Drug Intelligence and Clinical Pharmacy* (1977) 11:81–89.

MacNamara, M. "Talking with patients: some problems met by medical students." *British Journal of Medical Education* (1974) 8, 17–23.

McCloskey, J. "Influence of rewards and incentives on staff nurse turnover rate." *Nursing Research* (1974) 23:238–47.

McGhie, A. *The Patient's Attitude to Nursing Care.* Edinburgh: Livingstone, 1961.

Mettlin, C. and Woelfel, J. "Interpersonal influence and symptoms of stress." *Journal of Health and Social Behavior* (1975) 311–19.

Miller, D.; Brimigion, J.; Keller, D.; and Woodruff, S. "Nurse-physician communication in a nursing home setting." *Gerontologist* (1972) 12:225–29.

Moreland, J.; Ivey, A.; and Phillips, J. "An evaluation of microcounselling as an interview training tool." *Journal of Consulting and Clinical Psychology* (1973) 41:294.

Nelson, B. "The unpopular patient." *Modern Hospital* (1973) 121:70–72.

Norris, C. "Nurse and the crying patient." *American Journal of Nursing* (1957) 57:323–27.

Orvin, G. "Interviewing the adolescent." *Journal of the South Carolina Medical Association* (1970) 66:282–84.

Pacoe, L.; Naar, R.; Guyett, I., and Wells, R. "Training medical students in interpersonal relationship skills." *Journal of Medical Education* (1976) 51:743.

Parkes, M. "The nurse as a counsellor." *Nursing Times* (1973) 69:156.

Pavlou, M.; Hartings, M.; and Davis, F. "Discussion groups for medical patients: a vehicle for improved coping." *Psychotherapy and Psychosomatics* (1978) 30:105–15.

Pearlin, L. and Schooler, C. "The structure of coping." *Journal of Health and Social Behavior* (1978) 19:2–21.

Pueschel, S. and Murphy, A. "Counseling parents of infants with Down's syndrome." *Postgraduate Medicine* (1975) 58(7):90–95.

Quint, J. "Awareness of death and the nurse's composure." *Nursing Research* (1966) 15:49–55.

Raphael, W. "Do we know what patients think? A survey comparing the views of patients, staff and committee members." *International Journal of Nursing Studies* (1967) 4:209–23.

Raphael, R. "Patients and their hospitals." London: King Edward Fund, 1969.

Rasche, L.; Bernstein, L.; and Veen Huis, P. "Evaluation of a systematic approach to teaching interviewing." *Journal of Medical Education* (1974) 49:589.

Revans, R. *Standards for morale: cause and effect in hospitals.* London: Tavistock, 1964.

Robinson, A. "Professional conflict in the ICU/CCU." *RN* (1972) 35:40–45.

Robinson, L. *Psychological Aspects of the Care of Hospitalized Patients.* Philadelphia: F. A. Davis, 1968.

Sabshin, M. "Nurse-doctor-patient relationships in psychiatry." *The American Journal of Nursing* (1957) 57:188–92.

Santiesteban, A. "The use of psychological models in medical education." *Journal of Medical Education* (1975) 50:636–37.

Schmidt, D. and Messner, E. "The role of the family physician in the crisis of impending divorce." *Journal of Family Practice* (1975) 2(2):99–102.

Scoggins, J. "Communicate, dammit!" *RN* (1976) 39:38–41.

Scott, N.; Connelly, M.; and Hess, J. "Longitudinal investigation of changes in interviewing performance of medical students." *Journal of Clinical Psychology* (1976) 32(2):424–31.

Secundy, M. and Katz, V. "Factors in patient-doctor communication: a communication skills elective." *Journal of Medical Education* (1975) 50:689.

Sethee, U. "Verbal responses of nurses to patients in emotion-laden situations in public health nursing." *Nursing Research* (1967) 16:365–68.

Shocket, B. "The difficult patient in the general hospital." *American Family Physician* (1973) 7:95–99.

Skipper, J. "Child hospitalization and social interaction: an experimental study of mothers' feelings of stress, adaptation, and satisfaction." *Medical Care* (1968) 6:496–506.

Skipper, J.; Tagliacozzo, D.; and Mauksch, H. "What communication means to patients." *American Journal of Nursing* (1964) 64:101-103.

Smiley, O. and Smiley, R. "Interviewing techniques for nurses." *Canadian Journal of Public Health* (1974) 65:281-83.

Smith, K. "Forum: commitment to caring." *Image* (1969) 3(1): 15-18.

Sorenson, K. and Amis, D. "Understanding the world of the chronically ill." *The American Journal of Nursing* (1976) 67:811-17.

Spitzer, S. and Sobel, R. "Preferences for patients and patient behavior." *Nursing Research* (1962) 11:233-35.

Stein, R. "The student nurse: a study of needs, roles, and conflicts, part II." *Nursing Research* (1969) 18:433-40.

Stockwell, F. "The unpopular patient." *RCN Research Project*, Series 1, Number 2. London: Royal College of Nursing, 1972.

Taylor, M. and Berven, D. "An evaluation for teaching interviewing in multiple settings." *Journal of Medical Education* (1974) 49:609.

Truax, C. and Millis, J. "Perceived therapeutic conditions offered by contrasting occupations." Unpublished manuscript, 1971.

Ujhely, E. "Current technological advances and the nurse-patient relationship." *Journal of the New York State Nurses Association* (1974) 5:25-28.

United Manchester Hospitals. Patient satisfaction survey: 1968-69. Manchester: Patients' Services Committee, United Manchester Hospitals, 1970.

Waldon, J. "Teaching communication skills in medical school." *American Journal of Psychiatry* (1973) 130:589.

Ware, J. and Snyder, M. "Dimensions of patient attitudes regarding doctors and medical care services." *Medical Care* (1975) 13:669-82.

Ware, J.; Strassman, H.; and Naftulin, D. "A negative relationship between understanding interviewing principles and interview performance." *Journal of Medical Education* (1971) 46:620-22.

Warren, S. "Relationship between morale and communication among health center team members." *Canadian Journal of Public Health* (1978) 69:133-37.

Werner, A. and Schneider, J. "Teaching medical students inter-
actional skills: A research-based course in the doctor-patient
relationship." *New England Journal of Medicine* (1974)
290:1232.

Worby, C. and Babineau, R. "The family interview: helping patient and family cope with metastatic disease." *Geriatrics*
(1974) 29:83-95.

Wu, R. "Explaining treatments to young children." *The American
Journal of Nursing* (1965) 65:71-73.

References for Chapter 2

Berlo, D. *The Process of Communication*. New York: Holt, Rinehart & Winston, 1960.

Berne, E. *Games People Play*. New York: Grove, 1964.

Harris, T. *I'm OK, You're OK: A Practical Guide to Transactional
Analysis*. New York: Harper & Row, 1969.

James, M. and Jongeward, O. *Born to Win: Transactional Analysis
with Gestalt Experiments*. Reading, Mass.: Addison-Wesley,
1971.

Maslow, A. *Motivation and Personality*. New York: Harper &
Row, 1954.

Raths, L.; Harmin, M.; and Simon, S. *Values and Teaching*. Colum-
bus, Ohio: Merrill, 1964.

Sathre, F.; Olson, R.; and Whitney, C. *Let's Talk: An Introduction
to Interpersonal Communication*. Glenview, Ill.: Scott, Fores-
man and Company, 1973.

Simon, S.; Howe, L.; and Kirschenbaum, H. *Values Clarification:
A Handbook of Practical Strategies*. New York: Hart, 1972.

References for Chapter 3

Cautela, J. R. "Covert reinforcement." *Behavior Therapy* (1970)
1:33-50.

Christensen, C. "An interpersonal coping skills approach to counselling." Unpublished manuscript, Ontario Institute for Studies
in Education, 1978.

———. "Development and field testing of an interpersonal coping skills program." Unpublished manuscript, Ontario Institute for Studies in Education, 1974.

Kanfer, F. "Self-management methods." In F. Kanfer and A. Goldstein (Eds.), *Helping People Change*. New York: Pergamon, 1975.

Meichenbaum, D. *Cognitive-Behavior Modification: An Integrative Approach*. New York: Plenum, 1977.

———. "Self-instructional methods." In F. Kanfer and A. Goldstein (Eds.), *Helping People Change*. New York: Pergamon, 1975.

References for Chapter 4

Anthony, W. and Carkhuff, R. *The Art of Health Care*. Amherst, Mass.: Human Resource Development Press, 1976.

Carkhuff, R. and Pierce, R. *The Art of Helping III: Trainer's Guide*. Amherst, Mass.: Human Resource Development Press, 1977.

Carkhuff, R.; Pierce, R.; and Cannon, J. *The Art of Helping III*. Amherst, Mass.: Human Resource Development Press, 1977.

Egan, G. *The Skilled Helper: A Model for Systematic Helping and Interpersonal Relating*. Monterey, Calif.: Brooks/Cole, 1975.

Gazda, G. *Human Relations Development: A Manual for Educators*. Boston: Allyn & Bacon, 1973.

Gazda, G.; Wallers, R.; and Childers, W. *Human Relations Development: A Manual for the Health Sciences*. Boston: Allyn & Bacon, 1975.

Gordon, T. *T.E.T. Teacher Effectiveness Training*. New York: Wyden, 1974.

References for Chapter 5

Bennis, W. G.; Benne, K. D.; and Chin, R. *The Planning of Change*. New York: Holt, Rinehart & Winston, 1976.

Bernstein, D. "The modification of smoking behavior: an evaluative review." In W. Hunt (Ed.), *Learning Mechanisms in Smoking*. Chicago: Aldine, 1970.

Caplan, G. *Theory and Practice of Mental Health Consultation*. New York: Basic Books, Inc., 1970.

Havelock, R. G., *The Change Agent's Guide to Innovation in Education*. Englewood Cliffs, N.J.: Educational Technology Publications, 1973.

Rathus, S. A. and Nevid, J. S. *BT: Behavior Therapy—Strategies for Solving Problems in Living*. New York: Doubleday, 1977.

Schein, E. H. *Process Consultation: Its Role in Organizational Development*. Reading, Mass.: Addison-Wesley, 1969.

Schindler-Rainman, E. and Lippitt, R. *Team Training for Community Change*. Riverside, Calif.: University of California, 1973.

Stuart, R. and Davis, B. *Slim Chance in a Fat World: Behavioral Control of Obesity*. Champaign, Ill.: Research Press, 1972.

Watzlawick, P.; Weakland, J.; and Fisch, R. *Change: Principles of Problem Formulation and Resolution*. New York: W. W. Norton and Co., Inc., 1974.

References for Chapter 6

Alberti, R. E. and Emmons, M. L. *Stand Up, Speak Out, Talk Back!* New York: Pocket Books, 1975.

_____. *Your Perfect Right*. San Luis Obispo, Calif.: Impact Publishers, 1970.

Bach, G. R. and Goldberg, H. *Creative Aggression: The Art of Assertive Living*. New York: Avon Books, 1975.

Baer, J. *How To Be an Assertive (Not Aggressive) Woman in Life, in Love, and On the Job*. Scarborough, Ontario: Signet, 1976.

Bloom, L. Z.; Coburn, K.; and Pearlman, J. *The New Assertive Woman*. New York: Dell, 1976.

Bower, S. A. and Bower, G. H. *Asserting Yourself: A Practical Guide for Positive Change*. Reading, Mass.: Addison-Wesley, 1976.

Dyer, W. *Your Erroneous Zones*. New York: Avon, 1976 (See especially Chapter 3: "You Don't Need Their Approval").

Ellis, A. *A Guide to Rational Living*. North Hollywood, Calif.: Book Co., 1974.

Fensterheim, H. and Baer, J. *Don't Say Yes When You Want To Say No*. New York: Dell, 1975.

Galassi, M. D. and Galassi, J. P., *Assert Yourself! How to be Your Own Person*. New York: Human Sciences Press, 1977.

Gambrill, E. D. and Richey, C. A. *It's Up to You: Developing Assertive Social Skills*. Millbrae, Calif.: Les Femmes, 1976.

Lazarus, A. and Fay, A. *I Can If I Want To*. New York: William Morrow, 1975.

Phelps, S. and Austin, N. *The Assertive Woman*. San Luis Obispo, Calif.: Impact Publishers, 1975.

Rathus, S. A. and Nevid, J. S. *BT: Behavior Therapy—Strategies for Solving Problems in Living*. Garden City, N.Y.: Doubleday, 1977.

Smith, M. J. *When I Say No, I Feel Guilty*. New York: Dial, 1975.

Taubman, B. *How to Become An Assertive Woman*. New York: Pocket Books, 1976.

Wolpe, J. *The Practice of Behavior Therapy*. New York: Pergamon Press, 1973.

Zimbardo, P. G. *Shyness: What It Is, What To Do About It*. Reading, Mass.: Addison-Wesley, 1976.

References for Chapter 7

Anderson, N. "An interactive systems approach to problem solving." *Nurse Practitioner* (September-October 1978) 3:25-26.

Barrows, H. S. and Tamblyn, R. M. "Guide to the development of skills in problem-based learning and clinical (diagnostic) reasoning." Monograph no. 1. Hamilton, Ontario, Canada: McMaster University, (undated).

Benne, K. and Sheats, P. "Functional roles of group members." *Journal of Social Issues* (1948) 4:41-49.

Berner, E.; Bligh, T.; and Guerin, R. "An indication for a process dimension in medical problem-solving." *Medical Education* (1977) 11:324-28.

Bjorn, J. and Cross, H. *The Problem-oriented Private Practice of Medicine*. Chicago: Modern Hospital Press, 1970.

deBono, E. *Lateral Thinking*. New York: Penguin Books, 1970.

Faculty of Medicine. "Problem based learning in medicine." Educational Monograph no. 4. Hamilton, Ontario, Canada: McMaster University, 1973.

Feightner, J.; Barrows, H.; Neufeld, V.; and Nosman, G. "Solving problems: how does the family physician do it?" *Canadian Family Physician* (1977) 23:67-71.

Feinstein, A. *Clinical Judgement*. Huntington, N.Y.: Robert E. Kreiger Publishing Company, 1974.

Gordon, T. *T.E.T.: Teacher Effectiveness Training*. New York: Wyden, 1974.

Hauser, M. and Feinberg, D. "Problem solving revisited." *Journal of Psychiatric Nursing and Mental Health Services* (1977) 15:13-17.

Hurst, J. and Walker, H., editors, *The Problem-Oriented System*. New York: Medcom Press, 1972.

Kolb, D.; Rubin, I.; and McIntyre, J. *Organizational Psychology: A Book of Readings*. 2nd ed. Englewood Cliffs, N.J.: Prentice-Hall, Inc., 1974.

Kramer, M. *Reality Shock: Why nurses leave nursing*. St. Louis: C. V. Mosby, 1974.

McGuire, C. "Simulation technique in the teaching and testing of problem-solving skills." *Journal of Research in Science Teaching* (1976) 13:89.

Marshall, J. "Assessment of problem-solving ability." *Medical Education* (1977) 11:329-34.

Napier, R. and Gershenfeld, M. *Groups: Theory and Experience*. Boston: Houghton Mifflin Company, 1973.

Schmidt, H. *Problem-Oriented Education*. Department of Educational Development and Educational Research. Rijksuniversiteit Limberg. Maastricht, The Netherlands (undated).

Shulman, L. and Elstein, A. "Studies of problem-solving, judgment and decision-making: Implications for educational research." *Review of Research in Education*. F. N. Kerlinger (Ed.). Itasca, Ill.: F. E. Peacock and Company, 1975.

Simon, H. and Newell, A. "Human problem solving: The state of theory in 1970." *American Psychologist* (1970) 145-59.

Watzlawick, P.; Weakland, J.; and Fisch, R. *Change: Principles of Problem Formulation and Problem Resolution*. New York: W. W. Norton and Co., Inc., 1974.

Ways, P.; Loftus, G.; and Jones, J. "Focal problem teaching in medical education." *Journal of Medical Education* (1973) 48:565.

References for Chapter 8

Appley, L. A. "A current appraisal of the quality of management." *General Management Series No. 1526.* New York, 1952, American Management Association.

Aradine, H. "Interdisciplinary Teamwork." Nursing Clinics of North America, June 1970.

Arndt, C. and Huckabay, L. *Nursing Administration.* St. Louis: C. V. Mosby, 1975.

Barrett, J.; et al. *The Head Nurse.* New York: Appleton-Century Crofts, 1975.

Beckward, R. *Organizational Development: Strategies and Models.* Reading, Mass.: Addison-Wesley, 1969.

Browne, Joseph A. "Health professionals' participation at hospital ward meetings." Unpublished doctoral thesis, University of Toronto, 1977.

Claus, K. and Bailey, J. *Power and Influence in Health Care.* St. Louis: C. V. Mosby, 1977.

Dalton, G.; Barnes, L., and Zaleznik, A. *The Distribution of Authority in Formal Organizations.* Cambridge, Mass.: The MIT Press, 1968.

Hine, F.; et al. *Behavioral Science.* Boston, Mass.: Little, Brown and Company, 1972.

Marshall, V.; French, S.; and MacPherson, A. *Evaluation of a Psychosocial Program in a General Hospital.* Hamilton: McMaster University, 1974.

Rubin, I.; Fry, R.; and Plovnik, M. *Improving the Co-ordination of Care: A Program for Health Team Development.* Cambridge, Mass.: Ballinger Publishing Co., 1975.

Stieglitz, H. "Concepts of organization planning." In H. E. Frank (Ed.), *Organizing Structuring.* London: McGraw-Hill, 1971.

Tichy, Monique. *Health Care Teams: An Annotated Bibliography.* New York: Praeger Publishing Company, 1974.

Wise, H.; Rubin, I.; Beckward, R.; and Kyte, A. *Making Health Care Teams Work.* Cambridge, Mass.: Ballinger Publishing Co., 1974.

References for Chapter 9

Cannon, J. and Carkhuff, R. "The effect of rater level of functioning and experience upon the discrimination of facilitative conditions." *Journal of Consulting Psychology* (1969) 33:189-94.

Carkhuff, R.; Collingwood, T.; and Renz, L. "The effects of didactic training in discrimination upon trainee level of discrimination and communication." *Journal of Clinical Psychology* (1969) 8:104-07.

Cohen, J. "A coefficient of agreement for nominal scales." *Educational and Psychological Measurement* (1960) 20:37-46.

Downie, N. and Heath, R. *Basic Statistical Methods.* New York: Harper & Row, 1970. (See especially Chapter 7: "Correlation —The Pearson 'r' and The t Ratio or Student's 't'," pp. 178-85).

Ericksen, K. and Bluestone, R. Memo to the faculty. Ann Arbor, Mich.: Center for Research on Learning and Teaching, The University of Michigan, Oct. 1971, 46.

Gerrard, B. "The construction and validation of a behavioural test of interpersonal skills for health professionals." Unpublished manuscript, Department of Medicine, McMaster University, 1979.

Goldfried, M. and D'Zurilla, T. "A behavioural–analytic model for assessing competence." In C. D. Spielberger (Ed.), *Current Topics in Clinical and Community Psychology.* Vol. 1. New York: Academic Press, 1969.

Hoyt, D. "College grades and adult accomplishment." *Educational Record* (Winter 1976) 70-75.

Kent, R. and Foster, S. "Direct observational procedures: methodological issues in naturalistic settings." In A. R. Ciminero, K. S. Calhoun, and H. E. Adams (Eds.), *Handbook of Behavioural Assessment.* New York: Wiley, 1977.

Schwartz, R. and Gottman, J. "Toward a task analysis of assertive behaviour." *Journal of Consulting and Clinical Psychology* (1976) Vol. 44, No. 6, 910-20.

Appendix

ANSWERS FOR EXERCISE 1

WHERE IS THE PROBLEM?

Situation A: ☐ The patient has a problem.

The patient is very upset and cannot focus
on the task.

FACILITATION SKILLS would be useful in this situation.

Situation B: ☐ Task

The group was unable to stay on topic and
accomplish the task.

PROBLEM-SOLVING INTERPERSONAL SKILLS would be
useful in this situation.

Situation C: ☐ The health professional has a problem.

The health professional student was unable to
speak up when interrupted.

ASSERTION SKILLS would be useful in this situation.

Situation D: ☐ Task

The group was unable to decide how to
approach the task.

PROBLEM-SOLVING INTERPERSONAL SKILLS would be
useful in this situation.

Index